Dr Peter Rawcliffe graduated from Pembroke College, Cambridge, and carried out his clinical studies at the London Hospital in Whitechapel. He subsequently worked in the Gastroenterology Unit at the Hammersmith Hospital, London, and in 1979 moved to the Radcliffe Infirmary, Oxford. Here he was involved in research into coeliac disease, and in particular in trying to define more closely the damaging components of wheat gluten. He and Ruth James set up the Oxford Coeliac Clinic.

Ruth James gained an honours degree in nutrition from Queen Elizabeth College, London University, in 1975. Following State Registration, she became a dietitian in Oxford and developed a special interest in diets for patients with gastrointestinal disorders. She was Chief Dietitian for eight years at the Oxford Radcliffe Hospital.

THE ULTIMATE GLUTEN-FREE DIET

The complete guide to coeliac disease and gluten-free cookery

Dr Peter Rawcliffe, MA, MB, BChir

and Ruth James, SRD, MBA

Foreword by

A. M. Dawson, MD, FRCP
Physician to HM the Queen (1982–93)
Physician to St Bartholomew's Hospital, London

LONDON

This book is dedicated to Maggie Stopard

First Published in the United Kingdom in 1985 by Martin Dunitz Limited

Revised edition published by Optima in 1992
Reprinted 1994

Revised edition published by Vermilion in 1997

6 7 8 9 10

This revised edition published in the United Kingdom in 2004 by Vermilion, an imprint of Ebury Press
Random House UK Ltd
Random House
20 Vauxhall Bridge Road
London SW1V 2SA

Random House Australia (Pty) Ltd
20 Alfred Street, Milsons Point, Sydney,
New South Wales 2061, Australia

Random House New Zealand Limited
18 Poland Rd, Glenfield,
Auckland 10, New Zealand

Random House (Pty) Limited
Isle of Houghton, Corner of Boundary Road & Carse O'Gowrie,
Houghton 2198, South Africa

Random House UK Limited Reg. No 954009
www.randomhouse.co.uk

ISBN 9780091887742

Typeset in Sabon by SX Composing DTP, Rayleigh, Essex

Printed and bound in the UK by
CPI Mackays, Chatham ME5 8TD

Contents

Acknowledgements

We would like to thank Dr Sidney Truelove, Dr Derek Jewell, Dr Peter Sullivan, Dr Stephen Turner, Liz Todd and Julie Giblett for their helpful comments on the original manuscript. We also thank everyone else, including patients and local groups of Coeliac UK, who contributed recipes, or helped in other ways.

We are grateful to Nutricia Dietary Products for advice and for retesting some of the recipes and to Alison Dawson for her expert help.

We are very grateful to Sandra Nichols, Dietitian at the Oxford Radcliffe Hospitals NHS Trust, who has contributed to the 2004 revision; and to Dr Derek Jewell who has again kindly commented on a section of the present manuscript.

Last, but not least, thank you to Julia Kellaway and Imogen Fortes at Vermilion, for all their help and their unfailing patience.

Foreword

Coeliac disease is a well-defined condition in which wheat gluten causes damage to the absorbing area of the gut, so interfering with the nutrition of patients. It can cause a wide variety of symptoms, even though sometimes the gut manifestations are minimal. Keeping to a strict gluten-free diet can transform such patients' health which, in a number of cases, has been subtly impaired for many years before diagnosis.

But treatment does mean keeping to the diet. This book will help patients enormously to understand why this is necessary and how to prevent such a regime from interfering with their life.

There is an excellent explanation of how food is digested and absorbed and the nature of gluten and how it damages the gut lining. The main body of the book gives valuable hints on how a diet need not interfere with an active social life, both for adult patients and children. A great deal of advice is given about dietary requirements in general and, furthermore, how to make delicious food from gluten-free recipes, so helping patients to have a broad, varied and interesting diet.

All in all a good addition to the coeliac library: I advise every coeliac patient to read this admirable book.

Dr A. M. Dawson, FRCP *Physician to HM the Queen (1982–93), Physician to St Bartholomew's Hospital, London, and King Edward VII Hospital for Officers*

Preface to the New Edition

Since the first edition of this book in 1985 the world of coeliac disease has expanded greatly. From being a disease few people had heard of, coeliac disease has now come much more to the attention of the media and the public.

Doctors too have an increased awareness of the condition. Not only do they now have available good blood tests to help with diagnosis, but screening groups of people using these tests has brought about a realisation that many cases of the condition have been undiagnosed in the past. Patient-led groups, for example the excellent Coeliac UK, have also played a key role in increasing awareness of the condition and helping people with gluten intolerance: links with other conditions are receiving more attention and research has benefited from advances in immunology and genetics. A virtuous circle has been created.

So this seems an appropriate time for a new edition of this book; we hope you find it interesting and useful.

Dr Peter Rawcliffe and Ruth James, Oxford, 2004

Introduction

This book is for people who have coeliac disease – called celiac sprue or gluten-sensitive enteropathy (GSE) in North America – or dermatitis herpetiformis, and their families. Our aim is to help you understand your condition and to give practical advice on the gluten-free diet. The first part describes what coeliac disease and dermatitis herpetiformis are and explains the reasons for the treatment with a gluten-free diet. In the second part we give guidance on gluten-free cooking and over 100 tested recipes to help you enjoy an interesting and varied diet.

Two important notes
Firstly, this is not a fad diet book, nor is it intended that it should be used for do-it-yourself diagnosis or treatment. Many of the symptons of coeliac disease can occur in other diseases, so it is unwise to diagnose and treat yourself. You should instead seek qualified medical advice in the first instance. Apart from the fact that self-diagnosis and treatment might not work, you could be delaying the diagnosis of another, possibly serious, condition.

Secondly, this book can only offer general advice: what we say is intended as a general guide, not as individual medical advice. This should be sought from your family doctor or medical specialist, dietitian or other qualified adviser. We have tried to make this edition as up-to-date as possible at the time of publication, but medical knowledge and practice are changing all the time: your doctors will be in the best position to keep you up-to-date. Coeliac UK and equivalent organisations elsewhere also provide current information, including on-line (contact details are given on page 151).

WHAT IS COELIAC DISEASE?
Gluten, a protein found in wheat and certain other cereals, is harmless to most people. However, in coeliac disease it damages the small intestine and so causes a variety of symptoms. We do not fully understand why certain people are affected in this way.

First the anatomy and working of the digestive system. When food has been broken down by chewing, and swallowed, it enters the stomach. Here it is further broken down, both mechanically and chemically. The resulting soup-like liquid then passes through the duodenum and into the small intestine (see diagram below). The upper part of the small intestine is known as the jejunum. Further digestion goes on here and the food materials, which are by now well broken down, are absorbed through the intestinal wall into the bloodstream, and so distributed around the body. Anything that is not absorbed passes into the large intestine (colon) and is excreted in the faeces.

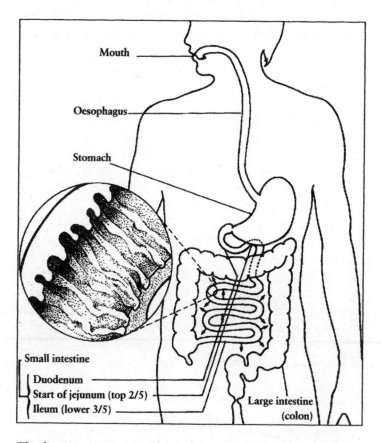

The digestive system; inset shows the circular folds of the small intestine, arrows indicate food being absorbed into the bloodstream.

The small intestine, then, has an all-important role in absorbing the food you eat, so that it can be put to use around the body. When it fails to work properly, and food is no longer absorbed normally, this is known as malabsorption. Coeliac disease is an important (but not the only) cause of malabsorption. Malabsorption of food results in weight loss and deficiencies of vitamins and minerals.

The small intestine under the microscope
The small intestine is a tube about 6.5 metres (20 ft) long and 4 cm (1½ in) in diameter. Its most remarkable feature is that its lining, called the mucosa, over which the food passes, is very highly folded. First, the tube itself has a series of large circular folds in its surface. Next, looking at the mucosa under the microscope we can see numerous finger-like projections: these are known as villi. Each villus is between 0.2 and 1 mm long and can just be made out with the naked eye.

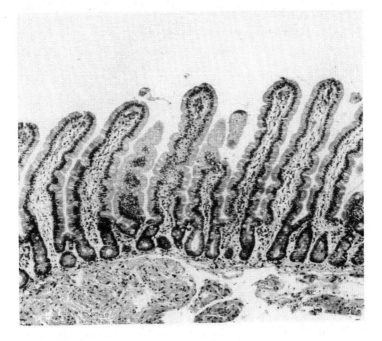

A cross-section of the lining of the normal jejunum with its long, finger-shaped villi (× 130). (In the duodenum the villi tend to be a little shorter, but are otherwise similar.)

A cross-section of a villus at a higher magnification shows a covering layer of tall cells (called enterocytes), and a central core containing, amongst other things, small blood vessels. Finally, if we look at the edge of a single villus at a very high magnification using an electron microscope we can see that on the surface of each enterocyte there is a regular array of minute projections (about 600 per cell): these are known as microvilli. Overall, because of all these foldings, one on another, the surface area of the small intestine is enormous. It has been estimated that the total area in an adult is about that of a tennis court!

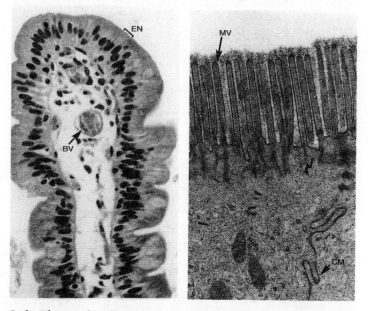

Left: The tip of a villus in cross-section (× 350); note blood vessels (BV) within and the enterocytes (EN) of the surface layer. Right: Part of a single enterocyte, showing the surface microvilli (× 20,000); MV = microvillus; CM = outer cell membrane.

During digestion the food particles are further broken down on the surface of the enterocytes before passing through the cells and reaching the blood vessels in the villi. From there they are transported away, in the blood, around the body.

In coeliac disease this process is upset because there is considerable damage to the mucosa, caused by gluten.

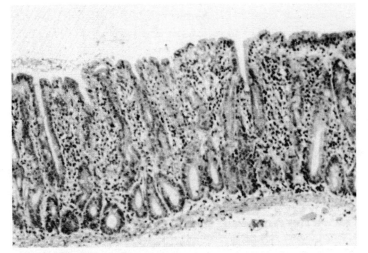

The intestinal mucosa of a patient with untreated coeliac disease. The surface is almost flat, with only the remnants of villi to be seen (× 130).

WHAT IS GLUTEN?

Gluten is a protein (or, more accurately, a mixture of many very similar proteins) that is found in several grain crops. The main source in the Western diet is wheat. The bulk of the wheat seed or grain, which forms the food reserve for the new seedling, is milled to produce flour. Flour has two major components – starch and proteins; the main protein is gluten. This is a very sticky material – the word gluten is a Latin one meaning glue, hence the adjective glutinous – and it is largely responsible for the excellent breadmaking qualities of wheat flour, giving it the characteristic doughy feel when mixed with water.

Some other cereals have similar proteins which, like wheat gluten, are also damaging to your intestine if you have coeliac disease. Rye and barley are certainly damaging but there is still doubt about oats (see page 37). Rice and maize are not harmful.

What effect does gluten have on the intestine in coeliac disease?

In coeliac disease the mucosa of the intestine is badly damaged by gluten. The villi are almost completely lost, only a few small bumps remaining. This appearance is often called a 'flat' mucosa and the villi are described as atrophic. Any microvilli that remain are shortened and irregular. Not surprisingly, the result of this damage, with the loss of healthy enterocytes and reduction of surface area, is malabsorption.

What are the symptoms of coeliac disease?

The damage to the intestine can lead to many different symptoms. The commonest are:

Babies and children	Adults
Miserable baby, crying and irritable	Weight loss
Failure to put on weight or gain height normally	Diarrhoea
	Anaemia
	Tiredness and weakness
	Abdominal discomfort and rumbling
	Recurrent mouth ulcers
	Sore tongue
	Bone pain (due to soft bones)

People vary greatly in the symptoms they have. Fortunately, not everyone has every symptom! Any pattern can occur: some people have one of the more unusual symptoms without having any of the commoner ones. None is characteristic of coeliac disease alone – similar symptoms can occur in other conditions. We describe later the tests that have to be carried out to narrow down the possibilities, and finally to decide whether or not someone has coeliac disease.

WHO GETS COELIAC DISEASE?

Both sexes are affected more or less equally, and both children and adults can develop the disease. Babies may begin to have symptoms as soon as they start on gluten-containing foods when they are weaned at about three to six months. The first appearance of symptoms is common from then on until 10 to 12 years old. It is unusual for the condition to start during the teens; most commonly it begins between the ages of 20 and 50. People can develop the disease even later – one of our patients in Oxford was 86 when she became unwell – though this is unusual. We do not know why some people are affected as children but others don't get symptoms until later in life.

How common is it?

Coeliac disease occurs in many parts of the world including Europe, North America and Australasia. It is quite common in Asians living in Europe. It is rarely diagnosed in India, Africa or China. There are probably several reasons for this. Dietary habits are different and people in these countries eat little gluten. Medical care is often less advanced than we are used to: people more readily accept ill-health and so the cause may remain undiagnosed. There may well be genetic reasons, too, with some races being less likely to develop the condition. Probably it is a combination of these factors, and maybe others we are not aware of.

Now that blood tests can be used to screen for coeliac disease (see page 18) it has been found that the cases of coeliac disease that are diagnosed are just the tip of the iceberg. (The figures that follow are very approximate but they serve to give an idea of the extent of the problem.)

Coeliac disease is diagnosed in one in 1,000 people in the UK. If undiagnosed cases, as suggested by blood tests, are included, the figure is about one in 100 to 200. Many of these people will have mild, or no, symptoms. If these undiagnosed cases are included, between 0.25 and 0.5 million people are likely to be affected.

The population of the EU in 2000 was 375 million. There are no overall figures for the incidence of coeliac disease in the EU but using the figure for the UK of one case in every 100–200 of the population (not an unreasonable assumption) gives a total of 1.8 to 3.75 million people affected.

A large-scale study published in 2003, using blood tests to screen for the disease, suggests that one in 133 people in the United States have coeliac disease – a total of over 2 million people.

Coeliac disease is particularly common in Ireland, especially on the west coast, where 1 in 200 to 300 people are actually diagnosed with the condition.

An inherited condition?

We have known for a long time that coeliac disease tends to run in families. Certain chemicals, called the HLA antigens, are carried on everybody's white blood cells and are known to be inherited – like the chemicals on the red blood cells which give you a particular blood group. Research has shown that these HLA antigens are found in a particular combination much more often in people with coeliac disease than in the rest of the population, so it seems that a person's genetic make-up is important in the development of the disease.

However, there have been a number of cases where only one of a pair of identical twins has developed the condition. As they are by definition genetically identical, there must be other factors apart from hereditary ones. A difference in the amount of gluten eaten is one possibility, but in many of the twins studied the intake has been very similar, so it looks as if there are other unidentified factors.

Although the way coeliac disease is inherited is complicated and not completely understood, some answers can be given to three practical questions that are often asked:

You say that coeliac disease is inherited. If that is the case why is it that none of my relatives has it?
This is not uncommon. There are several possible reasons. Firstly, you may simply not know enough about your relatives' medical histories. Sometimes when people go into their family history more thoroughly they do come across someone else with the condition. Secondly, there are undoubtedly people with a mild form of the disease who may never develop symptoms bad enough to take them to the doctor. This must have applied even more in the past than it does today. Again, minor symptoms may be attributed to other causes by the doctor as well as by the patient. Thirdly, we do know from careful studies done on several generations of families with coeliac disease, that the condition can skip generations. Finally, the condition has been known by other names in the past, including idiopathic steatorrhoea and sprue, so people may not realise that a relative has had coeliac disease.

What are the chances of my children having the condition?
If you or your partner have coeliac disease then there is approximately a one in 10 chance that any one of your children will have the condition. However, this may be an underestimate, if very mild and asymptomatic cases are taken into account (see How common is it?,

page 15). As coeliac disease is readily and effectively treated there is no reason for you to limit the size of your family on this account.

My child is perfectly well but is there any way you can tell whether he or she will develop coeliac disease later on?

The short answer is no. If there is coeliac disease in the family, particularly if either parent or a brother or sister has coeliac disease, you should, of course, make sure that your family doctor and health visitor or other medical attendant are aware of this. They can then be especially alert for any sign of coeliac disease developing. Many of the routine checks carried out at baby clinics are aimed at spotting anything going wrong at an early stage. If your child does develop any symptoms that cause you concern, discuss them with your family doctor or health visitor. Blood tests for coeliac disease are now available and can usually be arranged by your family doctor. This is discussed further on page 18. If necessary, your doctor might suggest getting the opinion of a hospital specialist.

In summary, if your child is well and growing normally there is no cause for immediate concern; but it is worth you (and, when they are old enough, your child) being aware of the possibility of coeliac disease in the longer term. See also the discussion on page 20 about whether well people should be screened for coeliac disease.

How is coeliac disease diagnosed?

Anyone who has already been diagnosed may prefer to skip this section. For readers who are beginning tests or who have a child being investigated we hope to give some idea about what is being done and why, and what you may expect. Every case is different, and the tests needed to exclude other conditions vary considerably. The tests also vary from one hospital to another, and are not always done in the same order. For these reasons this can only be a rough guide. If you are in doubt about what is happening, do not be afraid to ask: most doctors are much more willing to spend time explaining things than you may imagine.

Many diseases can be diagnosed without any special tests. The rash of chickenpox, for example, can usually be recognised as soon as it appears. The diagnosis of coeliac disease is inevitably slower. It starts with your first visit to your family doctor to discuss your or your child's symptoms. Your doctor will enquire further into your story asking about other symptoms, about your family and so on, and will usually examine you at this stage. As we said earlier, the symptoms of coeliac disease can be due to many other causes, some of which will get better on their own. Particularly if your symptoms are not too severe, your doctor may decide to wait and see whether this happens. If your symptoms persist, if they are very troublesome or if there are special clues, such as a family history, the doctor will next ask for blood tests to be done. Depending on what they show, your doctor may want to do more tests to narrow down the possibilities further, or may decide to send you to a hospital specialist.

Which specialist you see will depend on your main symptoms. If, for example, you are severely anaemic, you may see a haematologist (blood specialist), while you are likely to go to a general physician or a gastroenterologist (specialist in intestinal disease) if your main symptom is diarrhoea. Children normally see a child specialist (paediatrician) whatever their symptoms. Most people are seen in an outpatient clinic – your doctor will arrange for you to go into hospital only if you are very unwell.

The clinic will have a letter from your family doctor giving the main points of your story, and the doctor will go over these with you. You will then be given a general physical examination. You will be weighed and asked to give a urine sample. The doctor will tell you what the most likely causes of your symptoms are and which tests still have to be done before a final diagnosis can be made. You probably won't need to go into hospital. The tests vary so much according to the circumstances that it is not possible, neither would it be very useful, to describe them all here. They will certainly include further blood tests, including anti-endomysial and possibly anti-gliadin antibody tests. Ask about arrangements for the others – for example how much time you will need to take off work, whether you will have to come into hospital, or whether you will be able to drive home after a particular test.

You will be given a further appointment to be told the results. If coeliac disease is still a possibility, you will need to have a duodenal biopsy (see page 20).

Blood markers for coeliac disease
Three different blood tests are now used widely to help diagnose (or to rule out) coeliac disease. These are the anti-gliadin antibody, the

anti-endomysial (or endomysium) antibody and the anti-tissue trans-glutaminase (tTG) antibody tests. An earlier test, the anti-reticulin antibody, is less good and now not much used. The tests are not 100 per cent accurate – but figures of around 95 per cent (in some studies up to 98 per cent) for picking up coeliac disease are being achieved with the anti-endomysial and tTG tests. And (importantly) they only very occasionally (about 2 per cent) show a positive result in people who then turn out not to have coeliac disease on biopsy. (One of the reasons for differences in figures from different places is that if you set the test levels to try to make sure no cases of coeliac disease are missed, you tend to pick up more non-coeliacs in the process.) These figures are only to give you a rough idea, your doctor will know the figures for the particular test that you may have.

How are these tests used?

Where coeliac disease is clinically very likely, an intestinal biopsy will be needed. Extra blood tests are not likely to alter that and are therefore not likely to add much. But in many cases, where things are less clear-cut, blood tests can be very helpful. A positive test will suggest it will be best to have a biopsy; a negative test, particularly when coeliac disease seems fairly unlikely anyway, may avoid the need for a biopsy.

If suspicion of the condition remains despite a single negative test, one of the other tests can be done and/or the test repeated, or a biopsy may be decided on anyway. What is done will depend on the particular circumstances and will be matters for you to discuss with your family doctor or specialist.

The tests are used to monitor the response to going onto a gluten-free diet, usually going negative when the diet is strictly adhered to. (This is widely accepted though there does remain some dispute about it.)

Other conditions

Patients with insulin-dependent diabetes, some types of thyroid disease and some neurological disorders (and a number of other conditions) are more likely to have coeliac disease than people in general. A history of coeliac disease in the family increases the chance of someone having it. Anaemia, osteoporosis (see page 24) and infertility (Fertility and pregnancy, page 29; Fertility in men, page 31) can result from untreated coeliac disease, so, not surprisingly, patients with these conditions are found to have coeliac disease more often than the population at large.

Now that effective blood screening tests are widely available doctors are increasingly looking for (and finding) coeliac disease in these and other groups of patients. This has led in turn to a further increase in awareness of the condition.

Screening healthy populations

The tests have been used in surveys carried out to try to judge how common coeliac disease is in the population at large (see How common is it? page 15).

It has been suggested that the whole population of Europe and North America should be offered screening for coeliac disease – quite an undertaking if everyone accepted the offer! Whether detecting cases without symptoms would be worth the effort involved is not known. If genetic profiling becomes routine at some time in the future the situation might change. At present the best option is probably to screen people at particular risk, as mentioned above.

Duodenal biopsy

This is done with an endoscope in adults and in children. The endoscope is a flexible 'telescope' which can be guided down the throat (oesophagus) into the stomach and then into the duodenum beyond. Here a very small pair of forceps is used to take several pieces of tissue (biopsies) from the intestinal lining, the duodenal mucosa.

The endoscopy is done as a day case, that is you will be able to go home later the same day. In adults the endoscopy can be done without sedation if you wish. Many people though prefer to be sedated – by an injection – they are therefore not aware of the procedure and do not remember much about it afterwards. Babies and children are always sedated.

The tube is down for 5 to 10 minutes. If you have had sedation you will be closely observed afterwards until the sedation has largely worn off and you are awake again. You will then be allowed to go home. You may still feel a bit woozy at this stage and will certainly not be able to drive (or use machinery) for about 24 to 48 hours: the exact time depending on the sedation you have had. You will, therefore, need to have someone to collect you and take you home.

The biopsies will be looked at under a low power microscope and then sent for more detailed examination by a pathologist. Results are usually available in about 10 days. If coeliac disease is confirmed you will now begin your treatment with a gluten-free diet. To clinch the diagnosis your doctor will want to do further duodenal biopsies after you have been on the diet for about six months. This is to make sure that the intestine has recovered satisfactorily. In addition an antibody blood test will be repeated.

When there is still doubt about the diagnosis in adults a gluten challenge may be necessary. This simply means going back to eating gluten again after the second, improved, biopsy and then having further biopsies. If you have coeliac disease it will show damage again. A gluten challenge is very often necessary in babies and young children, but less often in adults: you must be guided by your doctor on whether you or your child need one.

There is no standardized procedure for the challenge in adults. Your doctor may ask you just to return to eating a normal diet; but he or she may ask you to eat a minimum amount of bread, say two or three slices each day, and sometimes to add gluten in powder form. Occasionally people get symptoms, especially of abdominal discomfort or diarrhoea, in the first few days of a gluten challenge. These almost always settle down within a week or so and the challenge can continue. Symptoms are less likely if you begin that challenge gradually, introducing a little more gluten each day over a course of a week, until you are back to a normal diet. As the challenge continues you may begin to develop symptoms again – for example, you may begin to feel tired, or your stools may become looser. The time it takes for this to happen varies.

To be sure of a clear-cut answer to the challenge, your doctor will arrange for biopsies to be done some weeks after you start it, unless you get troublesome symptoms beforehand, in which case the biopsy will be brought forward.

In children who are under two years of age when the diagnosis is first made, a gluten challenge is usually carried out later. The age at which this is done varies and will be for you to decide. This is to see what happens when gluten is eaten again. The usual gluten-free diet is continued (so good habits are not forgotten) but to this is added gluten in powder form.

An antibody blood test (see page 18) is done before eating gluten again and while eating it, and further duodenal biopsies are carried out while eating the gluten. Added gluten is taken for about three months or until the child gets symptoms which concern the parent, whichever is the sooner.

In children who are over two years of age when first diagnosed, a gluten challenge is not usually necessary as long as the first biopsy is typical of coeliac disease, there has been a clear-cut response to a gluten-free diet and the antibody test is initially positive and becomes negative on the diet. If in doubt, a challenge may be necessary, but in this case, a further biopsy is not usually carried out, only the antibody blood test.

How is coeliac disease treated?

In the second century AD, Aretaeus, a physician from Cappadocia (one of the eastern departments of the Roman Empire, today part of Turkey) who practised possibly in Rome, gave the first description of malabsorption. He also made some suggestions for treatment:

> In the first place, there is need of the juice of the plantain with water made astringent by myrtles or quinces. The stone of an unripe grape is also a very good thing . . . potions made with ginger and pepper and the fruit of the wild parsley which is found among the rocks.

Later authors gave similar descriptions, with even less palatable remedies. Robert Lovell of Oxford, England, writing in 1661, and quoting Pliny, says that 'the hee-goat spleen rosteth, helpeth the coeliack'. It was not until 1888 that, in his paper *On the Coeliac Affection*, Samuel Gee of London gave the first clear description of coeliac disease as a specific condition. Gee ends his paper with the comment that 'if the patient can be cured at all, it must be by means of diet'. He would be pleased to know how right he has been proved.

It was not until after the Second World War that it became clear what the diet should be. Dr W. K. Dicke and his colleagues, working in the Netherlands, noticed that children with coeliac disease, who had been making good progress under conditions of near starvation during the German occupation, began to do less well when wheat and rye again became available. During the next few years it was found that it was the gluten in wheat and rye that was harmful.

In 1954 Dr John Paulley of Ipswich in England noticed the atrophy of the villi in the intestines of people with untreated coeliac disease. A few years later it was discovered that the villi grew again when gluten was taken out of the diet, and that damage came back if gluten was reintroduced.

The treatment for coeliac disease is therefore a strict gluten-free diet. Gluten damages the intestinal mucosa whenever you eat it, and if you continue to eat it, symptoms develop. Even small amounts taken regularly can be enough to cause real damage. The sensitivity continues indefinitely so you will need to remain on a gluten-free diet for the rest of your life.

How quickly will I feel better on the diet?

Once you start a gluten-free diet the intestine begins to recover. The mucosa regrows and works normally again so that food is properly absorbed. This does not happen overnight; it will take several weeks or months for complete recovery. Some people begin to feel better almost right away, but in many cases it is three to four weeks before a definite change is noticed. A few people do not notice much improvement until six to eight weeks after starting the diet and this is especially true if you have been very anaemic. You will remain well as long as you avoid gluten.

What happens if I lapse on my diet?

If you eat gluten, the intestine will be damaged again and you will become unwell. In a study of adult and teenage patients from St Bartholomew's Hospital in London it was found that if they went back on to a normal diet severe damage to the mucosa developed in more than half within three weeks. In all the adults there was severe damage within seven weeks, though in some of the teenagers it took longer. There is of course mild damage much sooner. We know that gluten causes damage within a few hours of being eaten and repeated small amounts can add up to produce more severe damage. Symptoms are not a reliable guide to the state of the intestine as some people can have quite severe damage before they start to feel unwell. Therefore, while an occasional unintentional lapse is not a cause for alarm, you should not lapse unnecessarily. It is much safer to be strict so that your intestine is always working properly.

Other points

As we have already mentioned, coeliac disease can cause vitamin and mineral deficiencies. If these are marked when you are first diagnosed you may be prescribed an appropriate supplement until things are back to normal. In the case of most deficiencies, once you are established on the diet you will no longer need these supplements as you will now be absorbing enough from your food again. In the case of calcium and vitamin D things are more complicated and are discussed in the section on osteoporosis.

People with coeliac disease are more likely than other people to get a cancer of the intestine called lymphoma. However, this type of cancer is incredibly rare. And, if you stick to a gluten-free diet, you reduce the already minute risk still further. The chance of getting this condition is so small that no one should worry about it. (We mention it only to put it in perspective, in case people should hear of it elsewhere and worry unnecessarily.)

Osteoporosis

Osteoporosis is a common and a serious problem with one in three women in the UK thought to be at risk. While women are affected four times as commonly as men, men can also be affected. People with coeliac disease are more likely to have osteoporosis than other people.

Osteoporosis means thin bones (low bone density). Thin bones are more likely to break (fracture) even without any, or only minor, force. Hip, spine and wrist are bones often affected. Hip fractures are serious, and can lead to hospitalisation and major surgery. Spinal fractures can cause loss of height, severe back pain and deformity.

The causes of osteoporosis are several. They include an early menopause, lack of weight-bearing exercise, insufficient calcium or vitamin D in the diet, smoking, excess alcohol and a close family history of osteoporosis. There are other causes, but they are beyond the scope of this book. See page 151 for information on the National Osteoporosis Society in the UK.

Prevention is all – there is treatment but no cure for established osteoporosis. Obvious measures are not smoking and not drinking excessive alcohol. Sufficient calcium in the diet is important. Weight-bearing exercise (20 minutes, 3 times a week) such as walking, dancing or jogging, is helpful. If you are not in the habit of taking regular exercise you should discuss it first with your doctor and proceed gently.

There are other measures that can help. Hormone replacement therapy (HRT) in post-menopausal women is one, but there are potential disadvantages – the situation is in a lot of flux and this is very much an individual matter to decide with your doctor. Drug treatments are available for established osteoporosis.

Adults with coeliac disease are more likely to develop osteoporosis than other people. A failure to absorb calcium and/or vitamin D properly from the diet, at least before going onto a gluten-free-diet – in other words for years in many cases – seems likely to be a major factor. But once on the diet, people may eat less bread and cereals which are a good source of calcium (see page 37) and this may not help.

As well as the general measures above, what should people with coealic disease do? On pages 36–37 we discuss dietary calcium requirements and sources, including the possible need for calcium tablets. Vitamin D is also important for bones and supplements may be advised by your doctor. Coeliac patients, both men and women, should seriously consider having a bone mineral density (BMD) scan (also known as a DEXA or DXA scan). This is a painless and accurate way of measuring bone density. This is the only way of knowing whether you have the condition or not, other than waiting until you develop a fracture, which is too late in the day. There is some debate among experts as to whether having a scan is really necessary; in our opinion it makes a lot of sense to get this test done. We advise you to discuss this with your doctor.

If you have a child with coeliac disease bone strength develops up to the age of 30, so what happens in early life is important. Clearly a strict gluten-free diet will be very important. We advise that you discuss the question of osteoporosis with your child's paediatrician.

The National Osteoporosis Society in the UK has an excellent website. Publications, including one on coeliac disease and osteoporosis, are downloadable or available by post (see page 151 for contact details). There are similar organisations in other countries.

DERMATITIS HERPETIFORMIS

Dermatitis herpetiformis (called DH for short) is a very itchy rash that usually occurs on the elbows, shoulders, buttocks and knees, although it can appear anywhere including the face and scalp. It is not infectious. The spots are reddish and slightly raised and there are also small blisters that are easily broken by scratching.

DH is an uncommon condition which can affect both adults (most often between the ages of 20 and 50) and children, though the latter rarely. A survey from Edinburgh suggests that incidence in the UK is probably no higher than one in 20,000 people. It affects twice as many men as women. If you have a rash that may be DH, your family doctor will probably send you to a skin specialist. Diagnosis will include taking a small skin sample (biopsy) for microscopic examination. A local anaesthetic is given and the procedure takes only a few minutes.

What is the relationship to coeliac disease?

In 1966 it was found that many people with the DH rash had the same type of damage to the small intestine as is found in coeliac disease, although only about one-quarter to one-third of people with DH have intestinal symptoms, and these are usually mild. It is now known that about two-thirds to three-quarters of DH sufferers have a damaged small intestine, while in the rest it is normal. Though the damage can be as severe as it is in coeliac disease it is often less marked. As in coeliac disease, the intestinal damage is caused by the gluten and recovers when gluten is avoided.

There has been a great deal of controversy among doctors over how effective a gluten-free diet is in helping the DH rash, but most now agree that the rash does improve on the diet though it does not always clear up completely. If gluten is eaten again the rash tends to come back, though in a few cases this may not be for many months or even years.

We do not fully understand the connection between what happens in the intestine and the rash. Like coeliac disease, DH tends to run in families and both may occur in the same family. We know too that the HLA antigens on the white blood cells occur in the same pattern as in coeliac disease (see pages 15 and 33), all of which suggests a similar genetic make-up in people with these two conditions.

Treatment: diet or dapsone?

DH can be treated with a drug called dapsone. These pills are very effective and the itchy rash disappears, or at least is greatly reduced, often within a few hours and certainly within two or three days. You will probably be started on dapsone as soon as the diagnosis is confirmed. The next step is usually to carry out a duodenal biopsy (see page 20), particularly if you have any intestinal symptoms similar to those of coeliac disease, for example diarrhoea or weight loss. If the biopsy shows damage, your doctor is likely to recommend a gluten-free diet. If there is no damage, treatment with dapsone alone will probably be continued. You should use only as much dapsone as is necessary just to keep the rash and itching at bay, trying to reduce it from time to time. If you also start a gluten-free diet, you will gradually be able to cut down on the dapsone. Even if you are not on the diet the rash tends to come and go to some extent over the months and years.

You may wonder why everyone cannot simply take dapsone rather than go on the diet. For some people dapsone alone is a completely satisfactory treatment. There are, though, some possible drawbacks.

- To control the rash dapsone needs to be taken indefinitely. It can have various side effects, including damage to the red blood cells which may lead to anaemia. This is especially likely when large doses are being taken, in which case periodic blood tests may be necessary.
- One person in three or four with DH has intestinal symptoms or evidence on blood tests that they have malabsorption. Dapsone does not improve these symptoms or the malabsorption because it has no effect on the damage to the intestine.

The gluten-free diet can be a very useful treatment in such cases. It may take six months or more for the diet to be really effective, but by this time the dapsone can usually be considerably reduced, if not stopped altogether. Even when there is no evidence of damage to the intestine, a gluten-free diet may be worth trying, especially if dapsone is having any side effects.

There is one other drug that is sometimes used in DH – sulphapyridine. In general it is far less effective than dapsone but is sometimes used if dapsone is giving problems. Sulphapyridine can, though, also have side effects and a gluten-free diet is often a better answer in the long run.

You will have realised that the treatment of DH is not entirely straightforward. Every case has to be treated on its merits, and your specialist is the best person to advise you.

LIVING WITH THE GLUTEN-FREE DIET

After you have been diagnosed with coeliac disease or DH you should be seen by a qualified dietitian who will explain the gluten-free diet. Your doctor and dietitian will arrange to see you again in a few weeks' time. This is to check that all is going well and that your symptoms and blood tests are showing the expected improvement. Your dietitian may give you a number to ring him or her on if you have any queries about the diet between appointments.

Once you are firmly established on the diet and all the necessary biopsies are completed, you should keep in contact with the hospital clinic. If you move away, ask to be put in touch with a specialist in your new area. An annual outpatient visit is often all that is necessary. Blood tests will be done which will show up any deficiencies that may have arisen if you have lapsed, even unknowingly, on your diet. This visit also gives you a chance to raise any queries you may have with either the doctor or the dietitian. If you are worried about anything before your annual check is due, you can always arrange an earlier visit.

Children

Children will be seen at the hospital regularly, especially in the early years. Babies should also be seen by the family doctor and health visitor, usually at a well baby or child clinic, where they will be weighed to make sure they are growing normally, as they should on the diet. The weights are recorded so the baby's progress can be followed, and the measurements are best done at the same place each time. Older children should have their height measured as well. There is no general rule about how often these checks are necessary; it will depend very much on how the child is getting on, and the checks will be less frequent as the child gets older, but your doctor will advise you. On page 50 you will find practical points about the gluten-free diet for babies and children.

Teenagers

If you are a teenager you may find that sticking to the diet isn't always easy, especially if you have just been diagnosed. If you have had coeliac disease since you were very young it will be easier, as you will have learned how to cope with the diet over the years. As you are becoming more independent and away from home more and more, you may find it awkward and dull to stick strictly to your diet. Sometimes you may feel unwell soon after eating gluten – in a way this makes things easier as you will be less tempted to cheat. If you do not immediately get symptoms, you may find the temptation to cheat harder to resist. If, though, you are still growing (and most people go on growing until they are about 18), lapsing on your diet can cause sufficient damage to the intestine to slow down your growth. This is because you are not absorbing food properly and you may end up shorter than you otherwise would be.

In your late teens and early twenties you no longer run this risk as your growth will be complete. You may also find at this time that you can increasingly eat gluten without feeling unwell, although the intestine will still be damaged. If you do have occasional lapses during this time and do not get symptoms, you are unlikely to run into any problems or endanger your future health. Nevertheless, we are not advising you to ignore your diet, only if it is sometimes particularly difficult to stick to, you need not worry too much. In social situations you can avoid problems by knowing what alcoholic drinks you can have and what gluten-free snacks are available on the diet. See your doctor once a year so he or she can keep an eye on you.

Within the next few years you will probably lead a more settled life and will find it easier to return to a strict diet to keep you fit and healthy. If you want to have children this is especially important, as the chances of your having a child are reduced if you are not well treated on the diet – this applies to both men and women. And women who are well treated have healthier babies.

Fertility and pregnancy

Women who have had children after starting a gluten-free diet have shown increased fertility, easier pregnancies and healthier babies when compared with women having babies before being diagnosed.

Most women with coeliac disease, whether they are on a gluten-free diet or not, are able to have children. However, fertility is reduced in women not on a diet and, while miscarriage is not particularly common in women with coeliac disease as a whole, it is more common in those not on a gluten-free diet.

Antenatal care is available to all women to ensure that the pregnancy goes smoothly and to deal with any problems as they arise. You should let the midwives and medical staff know that you have coeliac disease. If you go into hospital at any stage of your pregnancy, please note the advice on page 49 about alerting the hospital that you need a gluten-free diet. Even though the doctors know you have coeliac disease, you will still need to ensure that the ward makes arrangements for your diet. Give as much warning as you can and check on arrival that the message has got through.

You must take particular care with your diet as the absorption of everything that you and the baby need depends on your intestine being healthy. You will feel better if you are on a strict diet. Women who do not stick to their diet often have diarrhoea and abdominal pain during pregnancy.

If you are newly diagnosed or have any concerns about your diet, you might want to think about taking a multivitamin/mineral supplement while you are pregnant. Discuss this with your doctor. It is important to get the right type of multivitamin tablet. Some have high levels of vitamin A; these should be avoided in pregnancy.

A special word about folic acid (folate). Folic acid supplements, 400 micrograms (mcg) daily, are now advised routinely in the UK and the USA during the first 12 weeks of pregnancy. Taking this extra folic acid has been shown to dramatically reduce the risk of neural tube defects (the best known of which is spina bifida) in babies. The practical problem that arises is that if you wait until you know you are pregnant before taking the extra folic acid, you will already have missed the all-important early weeks. The National Center on Birth Defects and Developmental Disabilities in the USA and the Food Standards Agency in the UK advise taking folic acid supplements anyway if there is any chance you may become pregnant (note that 50 per cent of pregnancies in the USA are unplanned). Women who have already had a child with a neural tube defect should consult their doctor for individual advice. In addition to the tablet supplements it is important to eat adequate amounts of folate-containing foods.*

If you have coeliac disease that is treated with a long-term and strict gluten-free diet then there is no reason to suppose you will be at extra risk of folate deficiency. However, it makes sense to be sure to follow the above advice, particularly because of the possibility of inadvertent lapses, or in case you have not been absolutely meticulous with your diet before becoming pregnant.

Blood tests are routinely carried out in pregnancy to check for anaemia. Anaemia is not uncommon in pregnancy and may sometimes be due to a shortage of iron, in which case your doctor may suggest you take iron tablets. If you have coeliac disease your doctor may additionally want to check your serum or red cell folate levels (blood tests), particularly if there is any doubt about how strict your diet is, or has been in the past.

Coeliac disease does not give rise to any particular problems with the birth itself. Babies born to well-treated coeliac mothers are, on average, of normal weight and as healthy as those born to non-coeliac mothers. Babies born to women with untreated coeliac disease on the other hand are, as you might expect, smaller than average. Provided your coeliac disease is well-treated there is no reason why you should not breast-feed.

The message is clear: stick to a strictly gluten-free diet and your coeliac disease should not affect your pregnancy. It is important that your diet should be well balanced as well as gluten-free (we discuss this on pages 35–44). Your dietitian or health visitor will be able to give you further advice.

Fertility in men
Coeliac disease sometimes causes infertility in men, and this too will improve on treatment with a gluten-free diet.

The Food Standards Agency says on its website:
Brussels sprouts, asparagus, black-eyed beans, spinach and kale are rich sources of folate. Broccoli, spring greens, cabbage, cauliflower, iceberg lettuce, parsnips and oranges also contain significant amounts, but folate is destroyed easily when cooked and tends to be lost in the water used for boiling. You can increase your intake of folic acid by eating foods that are fortified with it, for example some breakfast cereals.
[NB This website (www.foodstandards.gov.uk) is an excellent source of advice on foods in pregnancy and is well worth a look.]

Coeliac UK

We would advise you to join your national coeliac organisation. In the UK, Coeliac UK, founded in 1968, is run by and for people with coeliac disease and dermatitis herpetiformis. There are local groups throughout the country, which hold regular meetings. The services and publications of the organisation are available only to members (see Useful Addresses, page 151); there is no membership subscription but donations are welcome. Coeliac UK is now amalgamated with the Coeliac Trust, which funds research into coeliac disease. Similar organisations across the world provide similar services – see Useful Addresses, page 151).

Coeliac UK annually produces a useful booklet, *The Gluten-Free Food & Drink Directory*, which gives the brand-name foods that do not contain gluten. Coeliac UK automatically sends the *Directory* to all members – there is a small charge for this. A magazine, *Crossed Grain*, is produced three times a year and contains articles covering a wide range of practical and topical matters affecting people with coeliac disease and DH. For coeliacs who are registered as either blind or partially sighted, cassettes of *Crossed Grain* are available.

As products change it is important to keep the *Directory* updated on a monthly basis:

- Complete lists of deletions, additions and changes are available from the Coeliac UK office (large stamped addressed envelope needed).
- A recorded message is available 24 hours a day on 0149 447 3510.
- BBC2 Ceefax page 659 gives monthly changes to the *Directory* during the first week of the month.
- Visit the Coeliac UK website (www.coeliac.co.uk) and subscribe to their automatic e-mail update service where you will be automatically e-mailed *Directory* changes at the beginning of each month.

Life insurance

People with coeliac disease are usually dealt with fairly favourably by life insurance companies. The company will require as full a medical report as possible. They like to know how severe the disease has been and how long it has been well controlled on the diet. There may be a moderate increase in the normal premium in the early years, but this will be reduced as the disease comes under control. After four to five years of good health on the diet, the premiums will usually be the same as if you did not have coeliac disease. With this as a guide to what to expect, if you shop around, you should not have any problems in getting good terms.

RESEARCH

For many years, research into coeliac disease has tried to answer two main questions. First, what is it about some people that makes them react badly to gluten? Second, remembering that gluten is a mixture of many proteins, which particular bit or bits cause the problem? Research is coming up with some answers.

In one line of research particular cells, called lymphocytes, have been prepared from biopsies of the intestine in coeliac patients and grown on in the laboratory. (Lymphocytes are one of the types of white cell from the immune system. We all have them, in many different areas of our bodies.) Gluten is treated in the laboratory with chemicals called enzymes, which break it into small fragments (a process similar to what happens when it is digested in the body). The cells and the digested gluten are then mixed. What has been found is that some particular gluten fragments react much more strongly with the cells than others. The amino acid sequence of the active fragments has been worked out (gluten is made of proteins, which consist of large numbers of amino acids joined together). Whether some of the active fragments are more important than others remains undecided by these tests.

In other studies, in Oxford, coeliac volunteers ate gluten, and lymphocytes from their blood were tested to see how they responded. One particular gluten fragment seemed to react particularly strongly with these cells; this fragment may be especially important.

The next bit of the story concerns tests for particular chemicals (known as HLA antigens) on the white blood cells of coeliac patients. HLA antigens are rather like blood groups. Which HLA antigens you have is determined by your genes – you are born with them and they stay the same all your life. These antigens are involved with the immune system of the body; the antigens are present on the surface of immune cells and determine the way they respond to things, for example to infections – or in this case to gluten. The majority of coeliacs have either the antigen known as HLA-DQ2 or that known as HLA-DQ8. And – you may have guessed! – for the particular gluten fragments mentioned above to react strongly with lymphocytes the lymphocytes have to have either HLA-DQ2 or -DQ8 on them.

One more thing – the gluten fragments react very much better with the cells if the fragments are first treated with an enzyme called tissue transglutaminase (tTG), which is naturally present in the intestine.

Finally, in coeliac patients but almost never in others, antibodies against tTG are present in the blood (hence the test for coeliac disease – see page 18; anti-endomysial antibodies are in fact directed against tTG).

So, what seems to happen in coeliac disease is this. When gluten is eaten it is digested by the body in the usual way. The fragments produced are then acted on by transglutaminase. Some particular fragments react with lymphocytes which have on them HLA-DQ2 or -DQ8. This triggers off an immune reaction that causes damage to the intestine. Exactly how transglutaminase antibodies fit in is not clear. Withdraw gluten from the diet, the process stops and the damage is repaired.

This is not the full story. The genetics are more complicated; not only are other genes involved, but some cases of coeliac disease may perhaps be connected with one set of genes, others with a different set. And if you look at identical twins (who are by definition genetically identical), in a significant proportion where one twin has coeliac disease the other does not, despite both eating gluten. Other quite separate factors may be important too, for example the age at which gluten is first introduced into a child's diet, and whether a child is breast-fed or not. People have suggested that particular viral infections in early life may also play a part. There is still work to do.

The Diet

For someone just starting a gluten-free diet, the prospect may seem daunting. The aim of this chapter is to show that this need not be so, and that the practical difficulties can be easily overcome. Having someone with coeliac disease in the family need not disrupt the rest of the household. Many foods are naturally gluten-free and can be enjoyed by all. The recipes offer new and interesting ideas in gluten-free cooking and eating.

Gluten is a protein found in wheat, rye and barley (see page 13). Although most of us eat it every day, it is not essential to our well-being. There are many countries where gluten is not eaten and where cereals such as rice, maize and millet, which do not contain gluten, form the staple diet. A gluten-free diet can and should be a healthy diet.

The position of oats in the gluten-free diet has long been controversial (see page 37).

A HEALTHY DIET

Our bodies require a variety of nutrients. Fat and carbohydrate are the main sources of energy, and protein is essential for growth and the repair of the tissues. A healthy diet is one that contains sufficient amounts of each of the following food groups:

1) Bread, other cereals and potatoes
2) Fruit and vegetables
3) Milk and dairy foods
4) Meat, fish and alternatives
5) Foods containing fat and foods containing sugar
(See table, The Balance of Good Health, page 38.)

The key principles are to:
• Enjoy your food
• Eat a variety of different foods
• Eat the right amount to be a healthy weight
• Eat plenty of foods rich in starch and fibre

- Don't eat too much fat
- Don't eat sugary foods too often
- If you drink alcohol, keep within sensible limits
- Try to eat about five portions of fruit or vegetables a day

Vitamins and minerals, while only needed in relatively small amounts, are also vital to many of the body's processes.

WHAT CAN I EAT AND WHAT MUST I AVOID?

The table on page 38 shows the very large number of foods that are naturally gluten-free and which you can eat without any problems. If you look through the table you will see that many of the things you eat at the moment are included: the gluten-free diet may not be as bad as you first imagined!

You must avoid all food containing gluten. Remember that it can come from wheat, rye and barley, and possibly oats. Wheat flour is the main ingredient of bread and pasta and is used in cakes, pastries and biscuits. However, gluten is also present in many recipes in smaller amounts and it is often used in processed and convenience foods without this being obvious (see page 38).

Vegetarian

There is no reason why a coeliac cannot eat a vegetarian diet, although this restricts the choice of foods further. Using eggs, cheese, milk, possibly fish, as well as soya beans, textured vegetable protein (TVP), tofu and Quorn will widen your choice. For further information contact the Vegetarian Society, enclosing a stamped addressed envelope (see page 152 for contact details).

Calcium

Calcium is important for strong bones. Other factors are also important in determining bone strength: see Osteoporosis, page 24.

The recommended intake of calcium for adults with coeliac disease is 1,500 milligrams per day (normal adult requirement = 750 milligrams per day).

Try to get enough calcium by eating foods rich in calcium as shown in the following table.

Calcium guide

	Calcium content (mg)
1 glass (200 ml/7 fl oz) milk	250
1 glass (200 ml/7 fl oz) calcium-fortified orange juice	245
matchbox piece of cheese (30 g/1 oz)	216
small pot cottage cheese (125 g/4 oz)	82
small pot low-fat yoghurt (150 g/5 oz)	225
small can sardines with bones (100 g/3½ oz)	500
small can baked beans (150 g/5 oz)	80
2 slices white/wholemeal bread	66/33
1 orange	72

You may find it quite difficult to get the recommended amount of calcium in your diet even with the help of the list, in which case talk it through with your dietitian or doctor, who may recommend a supplement. Some gluten-free flour mixes and breads are fortified with calcium.

Oats

When you cannot eat wheat, rye and barley the question of whether oats are allowed becomes important. The position of oats in the gluten-free diet is controversial. Some doctors, however, believe that all coeliacs should avoid oats, and you must be guided by your own doctor and dietitian. Some people can tolerate them but if you cannot, it is probably best to avoid oats to begin with and then ask your dietitian or doctor what you should do next. If you have been advised that you may include oats in your gluten-free diet, it should be remembered that oats and oat products can be contaminated with gluten, and you should consult Coeliac UK's *Directory* for oat products which are gluten-free. (We have included some oat recipes later on in the book.) Very occasionally people have mild symptoms such as diarrhoea or a rumbling stomach which seem to be related to eating oats. When this does happen oats are obviously best avoided.

Processed and convenience foods

Many manufacturers use flour not only as a thickening agent but also as a cheap filling ingredient. Its use may be obvious, in fish fingers, pies and sausages, or more difficult to spot – in stock cubes, mixed spices,

The Balance of Good Health

	(1) Bread, other cereals and potatoes	(2) Fruit and vegetables	(3) Milk and dairy foods	(4) Meat, fish and alternatives	(5) Foods containing fat and/or sugar
What's included	Gluten-free cereals e.g. Cornflakes, Rice Krispies, gluten-free pasta, rice, beans and pulses.	Fresh, frozen, canned fruit and vegetables and dried fruit. Fruit juice. Beans and pulses can be eaten as part of this group.	Milk, cheese, gluten-free yoghurts and fromage frais.	Meat, poultry, fish, eggs, nuts, beans and pulses.	Margarine, butter, other spreading fats, cooking oils, oil-based salad dressings, gluten-free mayonnaise, cream, gluten-free chocolate, crisps, biscuits, pastries, and cakes, puddings, ice-cream. Soft drinks, gluten-free sweets, jam, sugar.
Important nutrients	Carbohydrate, fibre, some calcium and iron, B vitamins.	Vitamin C, carotenes, folates and fibre.	Protein, calcium, vitamins.	Protein, iron, B vitamins, zinc and magnesium.	Fat and sugar.
Recommendations	Try to eat high fibre foods where possible e.g. brown rice or high fibre gluten-free bread, jacket potatoes. Try to avoid: having fried food; spreading butter thickly; rich sauces and dressings.	Eat a wide variety of fruit and vegetables. Try to avoid: adding fat or rich sauces to vegetables (e.g. carrots glazed with butter) adding sugar or syrupy dressings to fruit.	Eat or drink moderate amounts and choose lower fat versions whenever you can e.g. semi-skimmed or skimmed milk, low fat yoghurts or fromage frais and lower fat cheeses e.g. Edam, half fat Cheddar.	Eat moderate amounts and choose lower fat versions whenever you can e.g. lean meat, grilled fish.	Eat foods containing fat sparingly and look out for low fat alternatives e.g. low fat spreads. Foods containing sugar should not be eaten too often as they can contribute to tooth decay.

What Foods Are You Allowed?

	Gluten-free foods – allowed	Check* – may or may not contain gluten	Gluten-containing foods – not allowed
Cereals	Gluten-free flour. Rice, ground rice, rice flour, potato flour, soya flour, split pea flour, arrowroot, cornflour, maize, sago, tapioca, buckwheat, millet. Soya bran, rice bran. Gluten-free bread, pasta, crispbreads, pastry, cakes, biscuits, puddings.	Oats, oat bran.	Wheat, rye, barley and foods made from them. Ordinary flour and flour products e.g. pasta, noodles. Wheat bran, wheatgerm. Semolina, bulgar wheat, couscous. Ordinary bread, pastry, cake, biscuits, puddings, pancakes, ice-cream wafers, ice-cream cones, cakes and pastry mixes, crispbreads, slimming breads and biscuits.
Breakfast cereals	Any made from corn or rice e.g. Cornflakes, Rice Krispies.	Baby cereals and infant foods Porridge oats, oatmeal.	Any made from wheat or rye, e.g. Weetabix, Puffed Wheat, Farex.
Puddings	Homemade puddings made from gluten-free ingredients. Gelatin, jelly. Rice, sago, tapioca.	Dessert mixes, ice-cream, mousses, pie fillings, canned milk puddings, infant desserts, custard powder, canned custard, cake decorations, cooking chocolate.	Proprietary sponge, pastry puddings. Semolina.
Soups	Homemade soups using gluten-free ingredients.	Tinned and packet soups.	
Sauces and seasoning	Homemade salad dressings and sauces using gluten-free ingredients. Gravy thickened with cornflour or a gluten-free flour. Bovril, Marmite.	Stock cubes. Gravy mixes and brownings. Savoury spreads, bottled sauces, chutneys and pickles. Salad dressings, curry powder, 'cook-in' sauces.	Sauces and gravies containing wheat, rye or barley.

*Check Coeliac UK's *Directory*.

What Foods Are You Allowed? *continued*

	Gluten-free foods – allowed	Check* – may or may not contain gluten	Gluten-containing foods – not allowed
Milk	All types.		Milk with added fibre. Oatmilk.
Milk products	Plain and fruit yoghurts. Fromage frais.		Muesli yoghurts. Yoghurts containing cereal.
Cheese	All varieties.	Cheese spreads. Processed cheese.	
Fats	Margarine, butter. Cooking oil/fat. Cream (fresh/soured).	Packet shredded suet. Low fat spreads. Synthetic cream.	
Eggs	Eggs.		Scotch eggs.
Meat	Fresh/frozen, all varieties including poultry, bacon, ham and offal.	Tinned meat, sausages, beefburgers, meat paste, pâté.	Meat pies. Any meat cooked with flour or breadcrumbs.
Fish/shellfish	Fresh/frozen, all varieties. Canned fish in oil, brine or water.	Fish paste, canned fish in sauce.	Any fish cooked in batter or breadcrumbs.
Vegetables	Fresh, frozen, dried, canned in water or brine, including potatoes and root vegetables.	Canned vegetables in sauce e.g. baked beans. Potato crisps. Instant potato.	Dishes including flour or breadcrumbs. Potato waffles, croquettes.
Ready meals and convenience foods	All brands need to be checked regularly.*	All brands need to be checked regularly.*	All brands need to be checked regularly.*
Nuts	Plain nuts.	Dry roasted peanuts. Peanut butter.	
Fruit and fruit juice	All varieties. Fresh, frozen, tinned, dried.	Commercial fruit pie fillings. Proprietary baby and infant fruits.	Pies and tarts.

*Check Coeliac UK's *Directory*.

What Foods Are You Allowed? *continued*

	Gluten-free foods – allowed	Check* – may or may not contain gluten	Gluten-containing foods – not allowed
Sauces and seasoning	Salt, freshly ground pepper, herbs, pure spices, vinegar.	Mustard, mixed spices and seasoning.	Packet stuffing mixes.
Sugar/preserves/ sweets	Sugar, jam, marmalade, honey, golden syrup, molasses, black treacle.	Lemon curd, lemon cheese, mincemeat. Other sweets and chocolates, Mars Bars etc.	Plain boiled sweets, liquorice and lollipops. Seaside rock.
Raising agents	Yeast, cream of tartar, tartaric acid, bicarbonate of soda, gluten-free baking powder (proprietary or homemade).	Baking powder.	
Flavourings	Flavourings and colourings.	Beef essence, chicken essence, milkshake flavourings.	
Communion wafers	Gluten-free communion wafers.		Ordinary communion bread and wafers.
Drinks	Tea, coffee, fruit juice, squashes, fizzy drinks.	Proprietary milk drinks, cocoa, drinking chocolate, vending machine. drinks, barley water, tomato juice, cloudy fizzy drinks.	Horlicks.
Alcoholic drinks	Cider, wine, sherry, whisky, gin, vodka, rum and other spirits, Martini and other aperitifs, liqueurs.		Beer including real ale, draught, bottled, homebrew, stout. Low alcohol beers and lagers.

*Check Coeliac UK's *Directory*.

An example of a day's meals

Breakfast   Rice Krispies with milk
                    Fruit juice
                    Gluten-free toast, butter and marmalade
                    Tea or coffee

Mid-morning   Tea or coffee
                    Date and nut square (page 126)

Lunch   Tomato soup (page 55) with gluten-free bread
                    Gluten-free bread toasted cheese sandwich
                    Maggie's salad (page 59)
                    Fresh fruit
                    Tea or coffee

Mid-afternoon   Tea or coffee
                    Seed cake (page 139)

Main Meal   Chilli Con Carne (page 74)
                    Boiled rice
                    Baked Lemon Delight (page 111)
                    Tea or coffee

Bedtime   Milk
                    Gluten-free biscuit

pickles, spreads, or ice-cream (see the table on pages 39-41). It is essential to check the label on individual products and you should avoid any containing the following:

barley	edible starch	semolina
bran	farina	vegetable protein**
bulgar or cracked	food starch	wheat flour
wheat	malt and malt	wheat bran
cereal binder	extract*	wheatgerm
cereal filler	modified starch	wheat starch
cereal protein	rusks	unless specified as
couscous	rye	gluten-free

*Malt and malt extract: many people with coeliac disease have no problem with these. A few, if they are especially sensitive, may be better to avoid them, particularly when large amounts are used – e.g. in some breakfast cereals.

**Textured vegetable protein (TVP) and hydrolysed vegetable protein (HVP) do not contain gluten, but if 'vegetable protein' is listed, avoid it. Quorn and tofu are gluten-free.

Remember, though, that manufacturers can change the ingredients of products, so check regularly.

Monosodium glutamate is a flavour enhancer used in many products. Although its name is similar it has nothing to do with gluten and you need not avoid it.

Coeliac UK produces a list of gluten-free manufactured foods which is updated every year (see page 32).

If you are unsure whether a product contains gluten then it is best to avoid it. If you want to know more about a particular food product, consult your dietitian.

Alcoholic drinks

Cider, wine, sherry, whisky, gin, vodka, rum and other spirits, Martini and other aperitifs, and liqueurs are gluten-free. Although spirits are made from grains including barley, wheat and rye, all protein is removed during distillation.

Unfortunately we cannot be definite about beer or lager. These are made from barley, and increasingly wheat as well, and both of these are harmful. The grain is broken down during fermentation, but not completely, and small amounts of protein have been detected in beers, lagers, ales and stouts – it is therefore safer to exclude them and choose another drink.

Medicines

A few medicines contain gluten. For over-the-counter medicines, ask your pharmacist. For prescribed medicines, check with your doctor. Sometimes it will be necessary to ask the manufacturer, as the information is not always readily available.

Communion wafers

Communion wafers contain gluten, but special communion wafers, suitable for people with coeliac disease, are available: see the Coeliac UK *Directory* or equivalent guide in other countries.

PREPARING FOOD AT HOME

Baking and breadmaking

Where wheat flour is the major ingredient in a recipe straightforward substitution with gluten-free flour does not always work. The main examples of this are breads, pastry, biscuits and cakes. For these, special gluten-free flours have been developed and special recipes are required. For this reason there are many baking recipes in this book and all have been thoroughly tested. As with all cooking, experience is important and you may not achieve your best results at the first attempt. As well as the recipes, you will find hints and tips at the beginning of each recipe section to help you become a skilful gluten-free cook.

The special gluten-free flours now available are the result of a great deal of development by the manufacturers and have been much improved in recent years. Cakes and biscuits made with them are very good indeed. It is only fair to point out, though, that while it is now possible to bake good and palatable entirely wheat-free bread it is still not like ordinary bread. This is not surprising, as it is precisely for its glutinous qualities that wheat flour is chosen for breadmaking, the gluten giving structure to the loaf. You cannot expect things to be quite the same without it.

Gluten-free flours are different from normal flour to bake with. They are lighter and 'squeakier', some more so than others. There is a variety available. Some already contain a raising agent (self-raising flours), others do not (plain flours). They may not specify on the packet whether they are plain or self-raising, so you will have to check the ingredient list to see if there is a raising agent (bicarbonate of soda, yeast, baking powder). Most gluten-free products are made from special gluten-free wheat starch but increasingly corn and potato starch are being used.

Many people enjoy making their own bread, but if you do not want to do this, ready-made gluten-free loaves are available, tinned or in a sealed plastic wrap. There are also bread mixes (white and brown) which provide a good, quickly made, gluten-free loaf. Gluten-free bread can be made very successfully in a bread-making machine (see page 90).

Other flours Potato, chick pea, soya, split pea, maize, rice, arrowroot, sago and buckwheat flours are free from gluten. They are available from health food shops.

Baking powder Commercial baking powders may contain gluten, so check, or make your own using the recipe on page 91.

Sauces
Flour is also used as a thickening agent, for example in soups, sauces, gravies and casseroles. Even these small amounts of gluten are enough to be damaging. Standard recipes can easily be adapted, replacing the gluten-containing ingredient with a non-gluten alternative. For instance, in a stew, while the meat and vegetables are naturally gluten-free, the stock (if made from a stock cube), white pepper, and flour used to thicken the gravy, are all possible sources of gluten. Using a gluten-free stock cube or homemade stock, freshly ground black pepper and cornflour is all that is necessary to make this dish gluten-free. A selection of recipes modified in this way has been included in this book and we hope that they will be particularly helpful to the beginner.

Availability of special gluten-free products
Gluten-free products are available in most European countries, North America, Australia and New Zealand. In several countries, including the United Kingdom, some products are available on prescription. In the UK these include bread, bread mixes, flour and pastas. Less basic

items, such as Christmas cake, breakfast cereals and biscuits, are also made but are not prescribable.

It is worth checking regularly what special products are available as new ones are added all the time. Your dietitian will be able to tell you.

Your dietitian will also be able to tell you which chemists carry a good selection of gluten-free products. They tend to be the large town-centre chemists, but smaller chemists' shops will usually be able to order products for you, especially if you go to them regularly. Gluten-free products can be bought from supermarkets and health food stores, by mail order and internet shopping.

In the UK people with coeliac disease are not, unfortunately, exempt from prescription charges. If you are not entitled to free prescriptions for another reason (your GP's surgery should be able to advise you about this), it will probably save you money to buy a Prescription Prepayment Certificate (PPC). As a rough guide, it will be worthwhile if you think that you will have to pay for more than five items in four months or 14 items in 12 months. Phone 0845 850 0030 to find the current cost of a PPC. You can buy one using a credit or debit card on this number, or on-line at www.ppa.org.uk. For payment by cheque or postal order get form FP95 from your pharmacy – the form tells you what to do.

Contamination

It is important that your gluten-free foods are not contaminated by others that contain gluten, e.g. with batter in the deep-fat fryer in fish and chip shops; or by sharing breadboards with users of ordinary bread.

SPECIAL GLUTEN-FREE PRODUCTS AVAILABLE

Biscuits – plain, sweet, savoury, rusks
Bread, sliced, unsliced, vacuum-packed or tinned; white, wholemeal, bread rolls; white/fibre, French bread, pizza bases and baguettes
Crackers – high fibre, crispbreads, cracker breads
Flours and mixes – ordinary, high fibre, cake mix, pastry mix, pizza mix
Pasta – macaroni, cannelloni, shells, spaghetti, lasagne, tagliatelle, penne, fusilli
Other gluten-free cakes, e.g. banana, fruit, date and walnut

Soya and rice bran
Baking powder
Crunch bars
Muesli
Semolina
Communion wafers

FIBRE AND CALORIES
Fibre
Unless you take care your gluten-free diet may be low in fibre (roughage). This is because most of the common sources of fibre such as wholemeal bread, some breakfast cereals and wheat bran also contain gluten. Fibre forms bulk in your diet and helps regular bowel action, so lack of it may cause constipation. It is easy to increase your fibre intake from other foods by eating plenty of fruit and vegetables; the skins are high in fibre so eat them whenever possible. Pulses, lentils, brown rice and nuts are also good sources of fibre.

Wheat bran cannot be used to give added fibre because it may be contaminated with gluten, but soya bran is gluten-free. Try taking about two heaped tablespoonfuls (30 g/1 oz) per day divided between two or three meals. Introduce it gradually over the course of a few days. You will see that soya bran has been included in some of the recipes in this book. It can be used in many other dishes too, for example sprinkled on gluten-free breakfast cereals or added to soups, stews and casseroles. It can also be added to gluten-free bread and incorporated into many baking recipes. It gives the finished product a speckled appearance but does not alter the flavour. With experience you will soon learn which recipes are most suitable for added bran. Rice bran is also available but is not very high in fibre (rice bran is 8–10 per cent fibre, soya bran 70 per cent fibre). Neither soya nor rice bran is available on prescription in the UK, but they can both be bought from chemists and health food shops. Make sure you drink plenty of fluid.

Calories
Most people gain weight when they start their gluten-free diet because food is absorbed more efficiently. This is often no bad thing if they

have lost weight as a result of their illness. Sometimes though, people find that they put on more weight than they would like. It is unhealthy to be overweight: several diseases, for example, high blood pressure, coronary heart disease and some types of diabetes, are commoner in people who are overweight. It is easier to avoid putting on too much weight than it is to lose it later.

If you do become overweight you will need to reduce your calorie intake. The quantity of calories you are able to eat and still manage to lose weight depends on your age, sex, height, occupation and how much exercise you take. Your dietitian will be able to give you advice on a target weight and what intake you should aim for. Here are a few tips to help you to lose weight:

1. Restrict foods that are high in calories, mainly sweet and fatty foods. Weight for weight, fats have twice as many calories as carbohydrate or protein. Not only is fat high in calories but there is evidence that in excess it has other harmful effects, for example, in causing heart disease. A few suggestions about reducing calories in your diet, and fat in particular, are listed here. You may also find a 'calorie counter' booklet useful.

   • Trim excess fat off meat and avoid frying
   • Use skimmed or semi-skimmed milk rather than ordinary milk
   • Use cottage, Edam, Gouda or other low fat cheeses
   • Use low fat spreads on bread and toast rather than butter or margarine
   • Use a sugar-free sweetener in drinks, in stewed fruit (add after cooking) and on breakfast cereals
   • Choose low calorie soft drinks
   • Drink less alcohol. Alcohol has almost as many calories as fat
   • Eat more fibre. Fibre fills you up without adding calories

2. Don't skip meals. Try to eat three small meals daily so you will be less tempted to eat snacks.

3. Exercise is good for you and will help to burn off calories. But be sure to start gradually if you have not been exercising regularly for some time. Do not rush into vigorous exercise straight away. If you have any doubts about how much you should do, consult your doctor. Brisk walking or swimming are good ways for most people to start.

4. Above all you will need motivation, willpower and perseverance. If you cannot manage to lose weight on your own then joining a slimming group might help you. The fact that you are on a gluten-free diet does not matter.

Calorie and fibre values are given with each recipe. You will notice that a fairly large proportion of the recipes are baking or pudding recipes. We have included these because they are the most difficult to make with gluten-free ingredients – but they tend to be high in calories. So if you have a weight problem you must be careful how much of them you eat.

EATING OUT

At work
If the kitchen at work can provide you with gluten-free meals, this is ideal. Otherwise you can either choose gluten-free foods from the ordinary menu or take your own packed lunch. Drinks from vending machines may contain gluten.

Restaurants and hotels
You can enquire in advance about the menu if you wish: you will find many chefs are pleased to help. If you cannot do this, try to eat where there is a wide choice available because you will have to choose 'safe' foods from the menu. For starters, soups are best avoided unless they are clear. For a main course, plainly cooked meats or fish without gravy or sauces are fine. Fish cooked in batter is not suitable. Salads are usually safe but be careful about any dressing and remember that processed meats may contain gluten. Many puddings such as pastries, sponge puddings, gâteaux, ice-cream, flans and cheesecakes contain gluten. Fruit, fruit salad, sorbets or cheese are all fine.

In hospital
If you have to go into hospital for any reason, let the hospital know that you are on a gluten-free diet. If the admission is planned in advance the hospital will normally ask about any special diet on one of the forms you will be asked to fill in prior to admission. When you arrive on the ward check with your nurse that the message has got through. If you should be admitted as an emergency let your nurse know about your diet as soon as you can. Smaller hospitals do not

always have stocks of gluten-free foods so take bread and biscuits with you. Not all staff will know about the gluten-free diet: if you are offered something which you think may contain gluten, query it, in case a mistake has been made.

Hotels

For an overnight stay, it's easiest just to choose obviously gluten-free items from the menu omitting, for example, sauces or dressings where in doubt. You may find it is worth taking a supply of gluten-free bread with you anyway – crackers and prepacked breads are excellent for this.

For longer stays you'll probably want to find out in advance whether the hotel can provide a bigger gluten-free menu: some do, some don't. Coeliac UK has a UK holiday list with holiday accommodation of all types where you can be sure of a gluten-free diet.

Flying

A special meal can usually be provided, but most airlines require several days' warning. Coeliac UK has advice sheets on airline travel and holidays abroad.

CHILDREN

Children with coeliac disease are otherwise perfectly normal and will remain healthy provided that they keep strictly to a gluten-free diet. With babies this is easy to ensure. Many prepared baby foods are gluten-free. Baby rice is gluten-free and is an ideal start if it can be mixed with the baby's usual feed, whether it is breast milk or formula feed. Formula milks available in the UK are gluten-free.

When best to introduce gluten to the baby's diet is unclear, even in families where there is no history of coeliac disease. In families where there is a history of coeliac disease it is equally uncertain: unfortunately, there is no clear evidence from research to help decide.

What to do then? The most usual time to introduce gluten into the diet of a baby in a family where there is a history of coeliac disease is between six and eight months. But exactly when to do so will depend on individual circumstances, so this is very much something you'd be best to talk over with your doctor or health visitor.

Gluten-free sausages, pancakes and pasta, together with gluten-free sauces and gluten-free batter, make acceptable additions to a toddler's diet and gluten-free snack foods such as potato crisps, wheat puffs, Rice Krispie cakes and gluten-free fairy cakes can also help. Children's paints and play-dough may contain gluten. As your child gets older he or she will learn more about their diet and start to manage it themselves. Fitting your child's diet in with the rest of the family as much as possible will help them not to feel different.

School meals
Discuss your child's needs with the school. Some schools may be able to provide a special gluten-free diet. In any case, schools are now offering a wider choice of food and if your child is old enough to know what to avoid, choosing a varied and safe menu may be reasonably easy.

Alternatively, your child could take a packed lunch. You could include cheese, cold roast meat or hard-boiled egg with salad, gluten-free crackers, or sandwiches made with gluten-free bread, plus fresh fruit or gluten-free cake.

Parties
There's no need for your child to miss out on parties! Let the people giving the party know as soon as you can what foods your child can and cannot eat. If you are giving a party, then all the food can be gluten-free.

School holidays, outings and courses
Give the organisers plenty of warning: tell them what is needed and send food lists. Give your child a supply of gluten-free bread and biscuits to take along.

The Recipes

WEIGHTS AND MEASURES

The teaspoon (tsp) measurement used throughout the book equals 5 ml and the tablespoon (tbsp) 15 ml; both are level. Australian users should remember that as their tablespoon has been converted to 20 ml, and is therefore larger than the tablespoon measurement used in recipes in this book, they should use 3 x 5 ml tsp where instructed to use 1 tbsp.

Calories (Cals) have been rounded off to the nearest 10, as have kilojoules (kJ). Fibre values have been rounded to the nearest gram.

Unless otherwise stated, all recipes are to serve four.

Keep to either the imperial or the metric measurements in a recipe. Gluten-free flours are more difficult to use than ordinary flours. Accurate measurements are very important: measure all ingredients carefully, especially the amount of liquid. Because flours vary, you may find that more or less liquid is needed than is stated in the recipe – always add a little at a time until the correct consistency is obtained. Liquids should always be measured at eye level. Use the type of margarine stated in the recipe. Treacle and syrup should be measured with a warmed spoon. Oven temperatures are given as a guide but ovens vary so adjust to suit your own. Use the stated size and shape of baking tin. This is particularly important for gluten-free baking as the flours don't have the same structural properties as ordinary flours and may need extra support. Non-stick baking paper is useful and is available from supermarkets and department stores. Rice paper is usually gluten-free, but remember to check.

WHICH FLOUR TO USE?

Where any flour will do we have simply put 'gluten-free flour'. Plain or self-raising flour has been specified where necessary. If you use a self-raising flour instead of plain, omit the baking powder and vice versa. Add 4 level teaspoonfuls of baking powder to 450 g/1 lb plain flour.

Not all plain gluten-free flours (or all self-raising gluten-free flours) have exactly the same properties as one another. Most recipes were tested with Glutafin flour mixes. In a few recipes where it is likely that only a particular brand-name flour will work well we have indicated with an asterisk which flour has been used in testing.

Freezing

Almost all gluten-free baked products freeze well. As they tend to go stale quickly it is best to freeze them soon after making. Baking the small amounts needed for one person is time-consuming and uneconomical. If you have a freezer you can bake more at a time and freeze what you do not immediately need. We have indicated in the recipes themselves the few that are not suitable for freezing.

Microwaves

Gluten-free dishes lend themselves well to microwave cooking – consult your microwave cookbook on cooking instructions using a similar recipe.

Basic recipes

Basic and other recipes given in the book and used within other recipes are indicated by initial capitals, to make for easy cross reference.

Soups

Tinned and packet soups may contain gluten. Homemade soups are good and satisfying. For convenience make in bulk and freeze in suitable portion sizes. Use gluten-free stock cubes or a homemade stock using any standard stock recipe.

GREEN PEA SOUP

Each serving: 220 Cals/900 kJ, 3 g fibre

1 medium onion, chopped
60 g/2 oz margarine
2 rashers back bacon, finely chopped
550 ml/1 pt gluten-free chicken or ham stock
225 g/8 oz fresh (shelled) or frozen peas
salt and freshly ground black pepper
chopped fresh parsley

In a saucepan, cook the onion gently in the margarine until it starts to soften and turn gold. Add the chopped bacon and fry for a few minutes more. Pour in the stock, add the peas and simmer gently until they are cooked. Liquidise or rub through a sieve and dilute to taste with more stock. Season to taste. Reheat, sprinkle with the chopped parsley and serve.

This soup is particularly good made with smoked bacon. Dried peas can also be used: 115 g/4 oz dried peas, soaked overnight, and the cooking time increased to 1 hour.

TOMATO SOUP

Each serving: 100 Cals/420 kJ, 3 g fibre

15 g/½ oz margarine
2 tsp olive oil
115 g/4 oz potatoes, peeled and diced
115 g/4 oz onions, diced
450 g/1 lb ripe tomatoes, skinned and roughly chopped
1 tbsp chopped fresh parsley
¼ tsp chopped fresh thyme
¼ tsp salt
freshly ground black pepper
1 tsp sugar
340 ml/12 fl oz gluten-free chicken stock

Heat the margarine and the oil in a large saucepan. Add the potatoes and onions and fry for about 5 minutes without browning. Stir in the tomatoes, herbs (reserving some parsley for garnishing), seasoning and sugar. Cook for a few more minutes. Pour in the chicken stock, bring to the boil, cover and simmer for 15–20 minutes until the vegetables are tender. Rub through a sieve and adjust the seasoning. Reheat and serve piping hot, garnished with the reserved parsley.

CREAM OF CELERY SOUP

Each serving: 240 Cals/1010 kJ, 4 g fibre

30 g/1 oz margarine
350 g/12 oz celery stalks, chopped
115 g/4 oz potatoes, peeled and cut into chunks
2 medium leeks, sliced
550 ml/1 pt gluten-free chicken stock
¼ tsp celery seed (optional)
140 ml/5 fl oz single cream or crème fraiche
285 ml/½ pt milk
salt and freshly ground black pepper
Garnish:
a dash of cream
celery leaves or fresh parsley, chopped

In a large pan melt the margarine over a low heat and add the celery, potatoes and leeks. Stir well, cover and cook for about 15 minutes. Add the stock with the celery seeds and a pinch of salt. Bring to simmering point and cook very gently for 25 minutes or until the vegetables are tender.

Purée the soup by liquidising or rubbing through a sieve, then return to the pan, stirring in the cream and the milk. Bring the soup back to the boil and season with salt and pepper.

Serve garnished with a swirl of cream and chopped parsley or celery leaves.

FRENCH ONION SOUP

Each serving: 490 Cals/2060 kJ, 2 g fibre

60 g/2 oz butter, plus a little extra
1 tbsp olive oil
450 g/1 lb onions, thinly sliced
2 cloves garlic, crushed
½ tsp sugar
825 ml/1½ pt gluten-free beef stock
285 ml/½ pt white wine or cider
salt and freshly ground black pepper
4 large croûtons gluten-free bread
170 g/6 oz cheese, grated

Heat the 60 g/2 oz butter and the oil together in a large heavy-based saucepan. Add the onions, garlic and sugar and cook over a low heat for 30 minutes, stirring occasionally until the onions have turned an even, golden brown. Add the stock and wine or cider, bring to the boil, cover and simmer for 1 hour. Season to taste.

Spread the croûtons with butter and place one in each of four flameproof soup bowls. Ladle the soup on top and sprinkle with grated cheese. Place under a hot grill and when the cheese is golden brown serve immediately.

Bacon and lentil soup

Each serving: 290 Cals/1220 kJ, 5 g fibre

115 g/4 oz (dry weight) green or brown lentils
1 tbsp olive oil
4 rashers smoked bacon, finely chopped
2 carrots, chopped
1 large onion, chopped
2 celery stalks, sliced
225 g/8 oz tin tomatoes
1 clove garlic, crushed
1.1 l/2 pt gluten-free beef stock
115 g/4 oz cabbage, finely shredded
salt and freshly ground black pepper
chopped fresh parsley

Wash the lentils thoroughly in plenty of cold water, and drain.

Heat the oil in a large saucepan and fry the bacon gently. Stir in the carrots, onion and celery, and brown carefully. Add the lentils, tomatoes, garlic and stock. Bring to the boil, cover and simmer gently for 50 minutes. Add the cabbage and simmer for a further 10 minutes. Season to taste and serve garnished with the chopped parsley.

Minestrone soup

Each serving: 260 Cals/1090 kJ, 4 g fibre

30 g/1 oz margarine
1 tbsp olive oil
60 g/2 oz streaky bacon, chopped
1 medium onion, finely chopped
2 celery stalks, chopped
115 g/4 oz carrots, finely chopped
2 tomatoes, chopped
1 clove garlic, crushed
salt and freshly ground black pepper
1.1 1/2 pt gluten-free stock
1 tsp dried basil (optional)
170 g/6 oz leeks, chopped
115 g/4 oz cabbage, shredded
1½ tbsp rice
2 tsp gluten-free tomato purée
grated Parmesan cheese

In a large heavy-based saucepan, melt the margarine and the oil. Add the bacon and cook for a minute before adding the onion, celery, carrots and tomatoes. Stir in the garlic and seasoning, cover and cook gently for 20 minutes. Pour in the stock, and add the basil, if using. Continue to simmer for about 1 hour. Add the leeks, cabbage and rice and cook for 30 minutes. Finally stir in the tomato purée and cook for another 10 minutes. Serve in warmed soup bowls, sprinkled with Parmesan cheese.

Salads and Salad Dressings

Salads are naturally gluten-free and are not fattening. But watch the dressings – not only are they usually high in calories because of the oil, but they may contain gluten. Recipes are given for making your own French dressing and mayonnaise at the end of this section.

MAGGIE'S SALAD

Each serving: 170 Cals/710 kJ, 2 g fibre

2 red eating apples, cored and sliced

6 celery stalks, sliced

60 g/2 oz walnuts, chopped

3 tbsp gluten-free French dressing (page 62) or gluten-free Mayonnaise (page 63)

1 clove garlic, crushed (optional)

Put the apples, celery and walnuts into a bowl. Add the French dressing or mayonnaise and toss to coat the apples and celery well.

The garlic may be included in the dressing.

SALAD NIÇOISE

Each serving: 280 Cals/1180 kJ, 2 g fibre

200 g/7 oz tin tuna fish

a few anchovy fillets (optional)

1 crisp lettuce

½ Spanish (mild) onion, thinly sliced

8 black or green olives

1 green pepper, seeded and sliced

4 tomatoes, quartered

2 hard-boiled eggs, quartered

8 radishes, trimmed

6 tbsp gluten-free French dressing (page 62)

Drain the tuna fish and flake roughly. Cut the anchovy fillets, if using, into 2-cm/1-in pieces. Tear the lettuce leaves and arrange in a bowl. Mix the tuna fish, onion, olives, green pepper and anchovy pieces together and place on the lettuce. Arrange the quartered tomatoes, eggs and radishes on top. Pour the French dressing over.

Hot gluten-free garlic bread goes well with this salad.

SUMMER PASTA SALAD WITH AVOCADO, APPLE AND MACKEREL

Each serving: 350 Cals/1460 kJ, 2 g fibre

225 g/8 oz gluten-free pasta spirals

1 avocado, peeled, sliced and tossed in lemon juice

1 large sweet apple, cored, diced and tossed in lemon juice

175 g/6 oz smoked mackerel fillets, cut into strips

3 spring onions, chopped

1 tsp whole grain mustard

salt and pepper to taste

cup-shaped lettuce leaves and grapes (optional), to serve

Sauce:

2 tbsp low fat yoghurt

2 tbsp gluten-free Mayonnaise (page 63)

2 tbsp crème fraiche

Cook the pasta for 6 minutes in boiling water. Drain and cool immediately under cold running water and put to one side.

Whisk together the sauce ingredients, add all the remaining ingredients, including the pasta, and lightly toss. Chill slightly then pile into cup-shaped lettuce leaves. Decorate with grapes, if using.

Pasta salad

Each serving: 230 Cals/970 kJ, 1 g fibre

115 g/4 oz gluten-free macaroni
200 g/7 oz tin tuna fish in brine
½ large cucumber, diced
2 large tomatoes, chopped
3–4 spring onions, chopped
4 tbsp gluten-free salad cream or gluten-free Mayonnaise
(page 63)
lettuce

Cook the macaroni as directed on the packet. Drain, refresh with cold water and drain again. Flake the fish into a bowl, add the macaroni and the other ingredients, except the lettuce. Toss, and serve on a bed of lettuce.

Kidney bean, courgette and mushroom salad

Each serving: 70 Cals/290 kJ, 5 g fibre

60 g/2 oz (dry weight) red kidney beans, soaked overnight in
plenty of cold water
170 g/6 oz courgettes, sliced
60 g/2 oz mushrooms, sliced
2 tbsp chopped fresh mint (optional)
1 tbsp gluten-free French dressing (page 62)
salt and freshly ground black pepper

Drain the beans and discard the liquid. Cover the beans in fresh cold water, bring to the boil, and boil for 10 minutes. Reduce the heat and simmer for 1¼–1½ hours or until the beans are tender. Drain and leave to cool. Steam the courgettes until just tender and allow to cool. Combine the beans, courgettes, mushrooms and mint, if using, and toss in the French dressing. Season to taste.

POTATO SALAD

Each serving: 330 Cals/1390 kJ, 3 g fibre

450 g/1 lb waxy potatoes, boiled and sliced
1 quantity gluten-free French dressing (below) or gluten-free
    Mayonnaise (page 63)
1 tbsp chopped fresh parsley
1 tbsp chopped fresh chives
4 spring onions, finely chopped
salt and freshly ground black pepper

Place the potatoes in a salad bowl, pour on the dressing and mix
thoroughly. Add the fresh herbs and chopped spring onions. Taste to
check the seasoning and keep the salad in a cool place until needed.

CUCUMBER RAITA

Each serving: 20 Cals/80 kJ, 0 g fibre

285 ml/½ pt gluten-free natural yoghurt
½ large cucumber, thinly sliced
salt and freshly ground black pepper
small clove garlic, crushed (optional)
chopped fresh parsley to garnish

Combine all the ingredients and garnish with parsley. Serve as a side
dish with curry (see Korma gosht, page 69; Vegetable curry, page 84).

FRENCH DRESSING

Each 15ml tablespoon: 100 Cals/420 kJ, 0 g fibre

6 tbsp olive oil
2 tbsp good quality wine vinegar
1 tsp gluten-free prepared mustard (optional)
1 tsp caster sugar (optional)
½ tsp salt
½ tsp freshly ground black pepper

Put all the ingredients in a bowl and whisk together using a fork.
Alternatively, put in a screw-top jar and shake vigorously. Any
chopped fresh herbs may be added. Store in the refrigerator.

MAYONNAISE

Each 15ml tablespoon: 100 Cals/420 kJ, 0 g fibre

¼ tsp caster sugar

1 tsp salt

1 tsp gluten-free mustard powder

3 tbsp fresh lemon juice

2 egg yolks

285 ml/½ pt olive oil

1 tbsp good quality wine vinegar

Into a warm bowl put the sugar, salt, mustard and 1 tablespoonful lemon juice. Add the egg yolks and, using a wooden spoon, beat thoroughly together. Drop by drop, add half the olive oil, beating well all the time. When the sauce is the consistency of whipped cream add another 1 tablespoonful lemon juice. You can now speed up the addition of the rest of the olive oil to a thin, steady stream – still beating continuously. Stir in the remaining lemon juice and wine vinegar, and lastly mix in 1 tablespoonful boiling water.

Keeps well in a screw-top jar in the refrigerator.

Fish, Meat and Vegetarian Dishes

Pure spices, fresh herbs and freshly ground pepper, invaluable additions to cooking, are gluten-free. But beware of ready-ground pepper, which can contain gluten. Take care with stock cubes and mixed spices such as garam masala and curry powder as they too may contain gluten. The quantities given in these recipes are usually for fresh herbs, but if you are using dried herbs, use about one-third of the amount stated.

Beans and lentils are included in several recipes. Because all beans and pulses are gluten-free and high in fibre they form a very useful and tasty part of the diet. They are high in protein and much cheaper than meat or fish, and since they contain negligible fat they are lower in calories. Dried beans, after their overnight soaking, must be boiled rapidly for 10 minutes before simmering until soft.

Rice is gluten-free. Brown rice has more flavour than white rice and more fibre, vitamins and minerals. When cooking any type of rice always follow the instructions on the packet. As a general rule use 1 cup rice to 2 cups water with a level teaspoon of salt. But some brown rice may need more water and take longer to cook.

Vegetables are also useful sources of fibre yet low in calories. They contain lots of vitamins and minerals. Do not overcook as this destroys a lot of the goodness. Potatoes are not as fattening as many people think, though adding butter to them when mashing, or cooking them by frying will greatly increase the calories. The skins are high in fibre, so scrub or scrape them rather than peeling and boil or bake them in their jackets.

Although meat and fish are naturally gluten-free, when they are cooked in casseroles or served with sauces or with gravy, you must take care not to introduce gluten – for example, thicken them with cornflour or gluten-free flour, as in these recipes, rather than with ordinary flour.

Meat is a good but expensive source of protein. However, even lean meat contains quite a lot of fat and so is high in calories. To reduce the fat trim off any visible fat and grill or braise rather than fry. Fish is less fatty, but again avoid frying – grill, steam, bake or boil.

Fish

HERRINGS IN OATMEAL

Each serving: 520 Cals/2180 kJ, 2 g fibre

4 herrings
salt and freshly ground black pepper
60 g/2 oz fine or medium oatmeal
60 g/2 oz margarine
lemon wedges

Ask the fishmonger to clean the fish and fillet them by splitting them down the back. Season to taste with salt and pepper. Coat both sides with oatmeal. Fry in the margarine until cooked through and lightly browned.

Serve garnished with the lemon wedges.

FISHERMAN'S PIE

Each serving: 400 Cals/1680 kJ, 2 g fibre

450 g/1 lb fresh cod or coley, skinned
salt and freshly ground black pepper
1 bay leaf
450 g/1 lb old potatoes, peeled
45 g/1½ oz margarine
140 ml/5 fl oz plus 2 tbsp milk
30 g/1 oz gluten-free flour
2 hard-boiled eggs, chopped
grated rind 1 lemon
1 tbsp lemon juice
¼ tsp cayenne pepper
1 tbsp chopped chives
1 tbsp chopped fresh parsley
30 g/1 oz Edam cheese, grated

Heat the oven to 190°C/375°F/gas 5.

Poach the fish in water, seasoned with salt, black pepper and the bay leaf, for 10–15 minutes. Drain and reserve 140 ml/5 fl oz cooking liquid. Boil the potatoes and mash them with 15 g/½ oz margarine and 2 tablespoons milk. Melt the remaining margarine in a saucepan, add the flour and cook for a few more minutes, stirring. Gradually stir in the remaining milk and the reserved fish stock. Bring to the boil, stirring continuously, to make a fairly thick white sauce. Flake the fish and add it to the sauce with the chopped eggs, lemon rind and juice, cayenne pepper, chives and parsley. Season to taste. Turn into an 825-ml/1½-pt pie dish. Sprinkle with the grated cheese. Spoon or pipe the mashed potato over the fish mixture and bake for 20–30 minutes.

BAKED STUFFED MACKEREL
Each serving: 330 Cals/1390 kJ, 6 g fibre

4 mackerel
salt and freshly ground black pepper
1 medium cooking apple
1 medium onion, finely chopped
60 g/2 oz gluten-free breadcrumbs
30 g/1 oz soya bran
2 tsp sugar
30 g/1 oz margarine, melted

Heat the oven to 180°C/350°F/gas 4. Grease an ovenproof dish.

Clean and bone the mackerel (the fishmonger will do this if you ask him). Sprinkle with salt and pepper and set aside. Core and grate the apple, mix with the onion, two-thirds of the breadcrumbs, and the bran, sugar, salt and pepper. Place some stuffing in each fish and fold over. Place in the dish, sprinkle with the rest of the breadcrumbs and pour over the melted margarine. Bake uncovered for 20–25 minutes or until the fish is tender.

SMOKED MACKEREL PÂTÉ

Serves 8
Each serving: 150 Cals/630 kJ, 0 g fibre

2 medium smoked mackerel
140 ml/5 fl oz soured cream
115 g/4 oz cottage cheese
juice ½ lemon
salt and freshly ground black pepper
pinch freshly grated nutmeg
pinch cayenne pepper
Garnish:
lemon wedges
watercress

Skin the mackerel and remove the bones. Flake the fish and put in a bowl. Add the soured cream, cottage cheese and lemon juice and beat with a wooden spoon until smooth; or place these ingredients in a blender and blend until completely smooth. Season, add the nutmeg and a little more lemon juice if necessary. Chill for several hours.

Sprinkle a touch of cayenne pepper on top and serve garnished with lemon wedges and watercress, accompanied by hot gluten-free toast.

KEDGEREE

Each serving: 410 Cals/1720 kJ, 2 g fibre

675 g/1½ lb smoked haddock
225 g/8 oz brown rice
85 g/3 oz margarine
1 onion, chopped
¼ tsp hot gluten-free curry powder
3 hard-boiled eggs, chopped
1 tbsp lemon juice
3 tbsp chopped fresh parsley
salt and freshly ground black pepper

Poach the fish in enough water to cover for 10 minutes or until cooked. Drain and reserve the liquid. Remove and discard the skin and bones. Flake the flesh and set aside.

Boil the rice in the reserved cooking liquid, adding water if necessary to make up the required quantity.

Melt 60 g/2 oz of the margarine in a large saucepan. Gently fry the onion until soft but not brown. Stir in the curry powder and fry, stirring, for 1 minute. Add the rice, flaked fish, hard-boiled eggs, lemon juice, parsley and remaining margarine. Season to taste. Warm through gently. Turn on to a warmed serving dish.

FISHCAKES

Makes 12

Each fishcake: 150 Cals/630 kJ, 0 g fibre

450 g/1 lb potatoes, boiled and mashed
450 g/1 lb cod or coley, poached, skinned and well drained
3 tbsp chopped fresh parsley
1 tsp gluten-free anchovy essence
1 egg, beaten
2 tsp lemon juice
a little freshly grated nutmeg
good pinch cayenne pepper
salt and freshly ground black pepper
For coating:
2 eggs, beaten
170 g/6 oz dry gluten-free white breadcrumbs
3–4 tbsp vegetable oil
knob of margarine

Mix together the main ingredients in a large bowl. Adjust seasoning. Refrigerate for an hour or so, until the mixture is firm. Turn on to a board dusted with gluten-free flour and lightly work into a roll about 5 cm/2 in diameter. Cut the roll into 12 slices. Dip each into the beaten eggs and coat with breadcrumbs. Heat the oil and margarine together in a frying pan and shallow fry the fishcakes until golden. Drain on kitchen paper and serve immediately.

Tartare sauce (page 150) or Parsley sauce (page 147) go well with these fishcakes.

Meat

MEAT FONDUE

A meat fondue can be prepared in the usual way – see any standard recipe book. If bread is to be included as well, you will of course use gluten-free bread. The following sauces are all gluten-free and suitable for both beef and lamb fondue: Tartare, Fresh tomato, Barbecue, Spanish and Curry sauces (pages 148–150).

KORMA GOSHT (MEAT CURRY)

Each serving: 290 Cals/1220 kJ, 0 g fibre

30 ml/1 fl oz olive oil
1 onion, sliced
2 bay leaves
1 stick cinnamon
8 peppercorns
8 cloves
4 cardamoms
450 g/1 lb lamb or stewing steak
4 cloves garlic, crushed
15 g/½ oz fresh root ginger, peeled and finely chopped or
    1 tsp ground ginger
1 tsp chilli powder
½ tsp turmeric
1 tsp ground cumin
1 tsp ground coriander
140 ml/5 fl oz plain yoghurt
salt
fresh coriander or parsley

Heat the oil in a large pan and fry the onion until light brown. Add the bay leaves, cinnamon, peppercorns, cloves and cardamoms and continue frying for 30 seconds. Add the meat, stir in the garlic and the remaining spices and fry, stirring, for about 7 minutes. Stir in the yoghurt, add 285 ml/½ pt of water, cover and cook over a gentle heat for 40 minutes. Add salt to taste. Garnish with coriander leaves or parsley. Serve with plain boiled rice and Cucumber raita (page 62).

BEEF CASSEROLE

Each serving: 410 Cals/1720 kJ, 5 g fibre

2 tbsp olive oil
450 g/1 lb chuck steak, cut into cubes
225 g/8 oz onion, sliced
1 heaped tbsp gluten-free flour
15 g/½ oz soya bran
285 ml/½ pt red wine or dry cider
1 clove garlic, chopped
2 sprigs fresh thyme or ½ tsp dried thyme
1 bay leaf
salt and freshly ground black pepper
115 g/4 oz field mushrooms, sliced
115 g/4 oz smoked bacon, cut into cubes

Heat the oven to 140°C/275°F/gas 1.

Heat half the olive oil in a large heavy-based casserole. Add the cubes of beef and fry to seal on all sides. Remove them as they brown and set aside on a plate. Brown the onion in the casserole. Return the meat, stir in the flour and bran and pour in the wine or cider, stirring well. Add the garlic, herbs and seasoning and bring to the boil. Cover the casserole, place in the oven and cook for 2 hours. Fry the mushrooms and bacon in the rest of the oil and add to the casserole. Cook for a further hour.

Steak and kidney pudding

Serves 8

Each serving: 430 Cals/1810 kJ, 4 g fibre

Crust:

225 g/8 oz gluten-free flour

½ tsp salt

115 g/4 oz gluten-free shredded suet

Filling:

225 g/8 oz kidney

675 g/1½ lb stewing steak, trimmed and cubed

2 tbsp seasoned gluten-free flour

1 medium onion, chopped

8 large mushrooms, trimmed

30 g/1 oz soya bran

dash Worcestershire sauce

First make the crust. Mix the flour, salt and suet together and slowly add sufficient water to make a soft dough. Roll out on a board dusted with gluten-free flour and line a 825-ml/1½-pt pudding basin, keeping back enough to make a lid.

To make the filling, toss the meat in the seasoned flour and put it with the onion, mushrooms and bran into the prepared pudding basin. Add the Worcestershire sauce and enough water to three-quarters fill the basin. Moisten the edges of the crust, put on the lid and seal well. Cover with buttered foil, pleated to allow the pudding to rise, and tie around the neck of the basin with string. Stand the basin on an inverted saucer in a large saucepan. Pour in enough water to reach halfway up the basin. Bring to the boil, cover the pan and simmer for at least 4 hours, topping up the water as necessary.

To serve, remove the basin from the saucepan, take off the foil and wrap in a clean cloth. Serve from the basin with a spoon.

QUICK PIZZA

This pizza can be cooked in a frying pan and finished off under a grill, or assembled on a baking sheet and traditionally cooked in an oven.

Serves 3–4

Each serving: 670 Cals/2830 kJ, 4 g fibre

Base:

175 g/6 oz Glutafin pizza mix

2 tsp gluten-free baking powder

1 tsp salt

2 tbsp olive oil

about 5 tbsp cold water

2 tbsp olive oil for frying

Topping:

125 g/4½ oz canned chopped tomatoes

pizza topping ingredients as desired, e.g. green or red pepper strips, gluten-free salami*, olives, anchovies, chopped pineapple, prawns, mushrooms, etc

115 g/4 oz cheese, grated

Heat the oven to 200°C/400°F/gas 6. Combine all the pizza base ingredients in a bowl and mix to give a soft dough, which can be easily handled. Turn out on to a surface lightly dusted with Glutafin mix and knead until smooth. Roll or pat out into a circle just large enough to fit the base of a large frying pan. Heat the extra 2 tablespoons of oil for frying and gently place the pizza dough in the pan. Cook gently on one side for about 5 minutes, then carefully turn over. Spread the chopped tomatoes and chosen toppings over the cooked side, finishing with the Italian seasoning and the cheese. Cook the other side of the pizza. Place under a preheated grill to melt the cheese. Or assemble the whole pizza, without frying, on a greased baking sheet and cook in a hot oven for 15–20 minutes until golden brown. Serve hot.

* Check your Coeliac UK *Directory* under *Sausages* for allowable makes.

Meat loaf

Serves 6
Each serving: 290 Cals/1220 kJ, 1 g fibre

2 large slices gluten-free white or brown bread
3 tbsp milk
450 g/1 lb lean minced beef
225 g/8 oz minced pork or gluten-free sausage meat
2 medium onions, very finely chopped
1 small green pepper, finely chopped
1 large clove garlic, crushed
1 tbsp gluten-free tomato purée
salt and freshly ground black pepper
1 tsp mixed herbs
2 tbsp chopped fresh parsley
1 egg, beaten

Heat the oven to 190°C/375°F/gas 5.

Remove the bread crusts and soak the bread in the milk. Squeeze out excess milk. In a large bowl, mix the meats, onions, pepper, garlic and tomato purée thoroughly together and season with salt and pepper. Add the soaked bread, mixed herbs and parsley and mix again. Bind together with the beaten egg. Press the mixture into a 1-kg/2-lb loaf tin and bake for 1¼ hours or until cooked. The meat loaf is cooked when it comes away from the sides of the tin. Allow to cool in the tin.

Serve cold, or hot with Fresh tomato sauce (page 148) or Quick tomato sauce (page 149).

CHILLI CON CARNE

Each serving: 460 Cals/1930 kJ, 23 g fibre

340 g/12 oz (dry weight) red kidney beans, soaked overnight in
   plenty of cold water
225 g/8 oz minced beef
1 tbsp olive oil
2 medium onions, chopped
4 tsp chilli powder
1 tbsp vinegar
1 tsp sugar
2 tbsp gluten-free tomato purée
140 ml/5 fl oz gluten-free stock
400 g/14 oz tin tomatoes
1 medium green pepper, seeded and chopped

Drain the beans and discard the liquid. In a large heavy saucepan, fry
the mince in the oil until browned. Add the onions and fry for a few
minutes until soft. Stir in the drained beans. Blend the chilli powder,
vinegar, sugar and tomato purée together and add. Pour in the stock
and the tomatoes together with their juice. Season to taste and stir to
mix well. Bring to the boil, partially cover and boil for 10 minutes,
then reduce the heat and simmer gently for 1¼–1½ hours, stirring
occasionally, until the beans are tender. Add the pepper 10 minutes
before the end of cooking.

PORK IN CIDER

Each serving: 450 Cals/1850 kJ, 4 g fibre

1 tbsp olive oil
4 pork chops, trimmed
6 rashers bacon
salt and freshly ground black pepper
5 juniper berries, crushed
2 cloves garlic, crushed
1 large cooking apple, cored and sliced
2 medium onions, thinly sliced
140 ml/5 fl oz cider
675 g/1½ lb potatoes, sliced
a little margarine

Heat the oven to 140°C/275°F/gas 1.

Heat the oil in a frying pan and fry the pork to brown on both sides. Remove and place in a shallow casserole. Lightly fry the bacon rashers and, using a slotted spoon, put on top of the pork. Season to taste: do not oversalt. Spread the juniper berries and garlic on top of the bacon and cover with the apple and onions. Pour on the cider and finish with a layer of overlapping potatoes. Dot with margarine, cover with foil and a tightly fitting lid and bake for 3 hours. Place the dish, uncovered, under a preheated grill to brown the potatoes. Serve immediately.

Frikadeller (summer pork burgers)

Serves 4–5
220 Cals/930 kJ, 2 g fibre

4 slices gluten-free bread
2 tbsp milk
450 g/1 lb lean minced or ground pork
1 onion, grated
1 tbsp finely chopped parsley
½ tsp ground allspice
1 egg, beaten
salt and pepper
30 g/1 oz Glutafin mix (any type) for coating

Cut off and discard the bread crusts and crumble the remains into a bowl to produce breadcrumbs. Add the milk and mix well. Stir in the rest of the ingredients. Use the Glutafin mix to lightly coat and shape the pork mixture into 4–5 rounds. Fry, grill, or barbecue the burgers until browned on both sides and cooked through, approximately 10–20 minutes.

STUFFED PEPPERS

Each serving: 280 Cals/1180 kJ, 5 g fibre

2 cloves garlic, finely chopped
2 medium onions, chopped
1 tbsp olive oil
340 g/12 oz cooked lamb or beef cut into small pieces
2 tbsp currants
salt and freshly ground black pepper
½ tsp ground cinnamon
½ tsp marjoram
400 g/14 oz tin tomatoes
4 red or green peppers
225 g/8 oz brown rice, cooked
4 tsp gluten-free tomato purée

Heat the oven to 190°C/375°F/gas 5.

In a frying pan, fry the garlic and onions in the olive oil for a few minutes, then add the meat and the currants. Season, add the cinnamon, marjoram and two of the tomatoes and 1 tablespoonful of their juice. Leave, uncovered, to simmer very gently. Meanwhile, cut off the stalk ends of the peppers and pull out the core and seeds. Rinse under cold water to remove all the seeds. Stand upright in a small casserole. Add the cooked rice to the meat mixture and mix thoroughly. Check seasoning. Fill the peppers with as much of the mixture as you can and put any remaining around the bases of the peppers. Top each with 1 teaspoonful tomato purée and pour the rest of the tinned tomatoes around the peppers. Cover the casserole and bake for 45–50 minutes or until the peppers are tender.

LAMB STEW WITH DUMPLINGS

Each serving of stew: 450 Cals/1930 kJ, 5 g fibre
8 dumplings, each: 130 Cals/550 kJ, 1 g fibre

1 kg/2 lb lean stewing mutton or lamb
5 tbsp seasoned gluten-free flour
340 g/12 oz onions, sliced
225 g/8 oz carrots, sliced
2 medium leeks, sliced
2 large potatoes, sliced
salt and freshly ground black pepper
2 tbsp chopped fresh parsley or mixed herbs
Dumplings:
85 g/3 oz plain gluten-free flour
1 tsp gluten-free baking powder
¼ tsp salt
15 g/½ oz soya bran
30 g/1 oz hard margarine
2 tbsp chopped fresh parsley

Trim the meat, remove any excess fat and cut into cubes. Coat in seasoned flour. Put a layer in a large saucepan followed by a layer of onion, carrot, leek and potato; season each layer with salt and pepper. Continue with the layers until everything is used. Add 1.1 l/2 pt hot water, bring to the boil, skim off any surface scum, cover tightly and simmer gently for about 2 hours.

Fifteen minutes before the end of cooking time make the dumplings. Sift the gluten-free flour, baking powder and salt into a bowl. Mix in the bran. Rub in the fat, add the herbs and mix to a soft dough with 4–5 tablespoonfuls of cold water. With floured hands divide the dough into eight balls.

Transfer the meat and vegetables to a heated serving dish and keep warm. Taste the liquid in the pan and adjust the seasoning. Bring to the boil and add more water or stock, if necessary. Drop in the dumplings, cover and simmer for about 15 minutes.

Arrange the dumplings around the meat and vegetables on the serving dish, pour over some of the liquid and serve immediately.

CHICKEN WITH MUSHROOMS AND BUTTER BEANS

Each serving: 330 Cals/1390 kJ, 10 g fibre

170 g/6 oz (dry weight) butter beans
2 tbsp olive oil
1 small onion, finely chopped
115 g/4 oz button mushrooms, sliced
½ small green pepper, sliced
½ small red pepper, sliced
225 g/8 oz cooked chicken
3 tbsp sherry
2 tbsp top of the milk
salt and freshly ground black pepper
1 quantity White sauce (page 147)
chopped fresh parsley

Soak the butter beans overnight in plenty of cold water. Drain, add fresh water to cover, bring to the boil, reduce the heat, cover and simmer for 2 hours or until tender. Add more water during the cooking if necessary.

Heat the oil in a large saucepan and gently fry the onion, mushrooms and peppers until soft but not brown. Cut the chicken into small pieces and add to the pan. Pour in the sherry and the top of the milk and season. Bring to the boil, partially cover and simmer for 3 minutes. Drain the cooked butter beans and add to the chicken mixture. Make the white sauce and stir it into the chicken mixture. Reheat and garnish with chopped parsley. Serve with plain boiled rice.

Spicy Thai chicken

Each serving: 290 Cals/1220 kJ, 3 g fibre

2 small fresh red chillies
60 g/2 oz onions
1½ level tsp lime rind, grated
1 stalk lemon grass
handful fresh coriander leaves
1 cm/½ in fresh root ginger, peeled
2 tsp lime juice
200 ml/7 fl oz white wine
salt and freshly ground black pepper
4 chicken breasts
2 tbsp olive oil
285 ml/½ pt double cream
1 level tsp sugar or honey
chopped red chillies
lime and coriander to garnish

Deseed the fresh red chillies and chop the onions. Place the chillies, lime rind, lemon grass, coriander, ginger, lime juice and 50 ml/2 fl oz of the wine in a food processor and whiz until smooth. Alternatively, crush the ingredients with a pestle and mortar. Season the chicken. Heat half the oil in a frying pan and fry the chicken for 4 minutes, or until crisp. Then fry the other side and set aside in a warm oven.

Wipe out the pan, add the remaining oil and fry the onions for 1 minute. Add the chilli paste and cook for a further 2 minutes. Pour in the remaining wine, bring to the boil and cook, stirring, until syrupy. Stir in the cream and cook for a further 2 minutes, sweeten with sugar or honey, add the chopped chillies and adjust the seasoning.

Pour the sauce around the chicken and garnish with lime and coriander. Serve with asparagus, broccoli and baby sweetcorn.

CREAMY CHICKEN PASTA

Serves 2

570 Cals/2370 kJ, 2 g fibre

140 g/5 oz gluten-free pasta spirals or macaroni penne
2 tbsp olive oil
½ tsp salt
285 g/10 oz chicken, cut into small pieces
1 onion, chopped
1 clove garlic, finely chopped
½ green pepper, chopped
½ red pepper, chopped
60 g/2 oz mushrooms, sliced
Sauce:
140 ml/5 fl oz single cream
pinch paprika pepper
pinch mixed herbs
1 tbsp gluten-free tomato purée
salt and freshly ground pepper

Cook the pasta in a large saucepan of boiling water with half the oil and salt for 7 minutes, stirring occasionally. Do not overcook. Meanwhile, fry the chicken in the remaining oil, add the onion, garlic, peppers and mushrooms and continue to sauté the chicken until it has changed colour and the vegetables have softened. Add all the sauce ingredients to the chicken and vegetables and simmer for about 5 minutes. Add the drained pasta and gently mix together.

Serve hot with Sun-dried tomato bread (page 93) and a fresh tomato and basil salad.

JACKET POTATOES

Choose large even-sized old potatoes, scrub them and prick several times with a fork. Bake in a hot oven, 200°C/400°F/gas 6 for 1½ hours or longer. When cooked they should be soft when squeezed. Cut open lengthwise and serve with a knob of butter, salt and freshly ground black pepper or one or more of the following fillings (quantities for 4 potatoes). Each potato, with filling:

115 g/4 oz Edam cheese, grated   *200 Cals/820 kJ, 3 g fibre*

200 g/7 oz bacon, chopped and
grilled   *350 Cals/1470 kJ, 3 g fibre*

200 g/7 oz tin tuna, with 1 tbsp
chopped fresh parsley   *230 Cals/970 kJ, 3 g fibre*

115 g/4 oz ham, diced, with
200 g/7 oz sweetcorn   *210 Cals/880 kJ, 5 g fibre*

Vegetarian Dishes

BUTTER BEAN CASSEROLE

Each serving: 290 Cals/1220 kJ, 13 g fibre

225 g/8 oz (dry weight) butter beans, soaked in plenty of cold
   water overnight
400 g/14 oz tin tomatoes
1 small onion, chopped
½ green pepper, chopped
salt and freshly ground black pepper
60 g/2 oz Cheddar cheese, grated

Heat the oven to 180°C/350°F/gas 4.

Drain the beans and put them into a casserole with the tomatoes, onion and green pepper. Season to taste. Cover and cook for about 2 hours or until the beans are tender. Uncover the casserole, sprinkle the cheese over the top and cook for a further 15 minutes.

MEDITERRANEAN BAKED COURGETTES

Serves 8
Each serving: 130 Cals/540 kJ, 2 g fibre

1 onion, chopped
3 tbsp olive oil
3 red or green peppers, seeded and diced
2 cloves garlic, crushed
8 courgettes, trimmed
salt and freshly ground black pepper
lemon juice
170 g/6 oz Edam cheese, grated
60 g/2 oz tin anchovy fillets

Heat the oven to 200°C/400°F/gas 6. Butter a baking dish.

In a frying pan, fry the onion gently in the oil until soft but not brown. Add the chopped peppers and garlic and cook for a further 10 minutes. Bring a large pan of salted water to the boil and cook the courgettes for 8 minutes. Drain the courgettes, allow to cool, and cut in half along their length. Using a teaspoon, scoop out a channel about 1 cm/½ in deep along each half courgette. Chop this flesh, add to the pepper mixture and cook for a few more minutes. Put the courgettes in the baking dish and season with salt and pepper and a squeeze of lemon juice. Fill each courgette with the pepper mixture; top with grated cheese and a strip of anchovy fillet. Bake for 30 minutes or until browned. Serve hot.

LENTIL ROAST

Each serving: 460 Cals/1930 kJ, 9 g fibre

225 g/8 oz (dry weight) red or brown lentils, washed (soak brown lentils overnight)

1 large onion, chopped

60 g/2 oz margarine

3 tomatoes, chopped

60 g/2 oz cornflakes, crushed

115 g/4 oz Cheddar cheese, grated

salt and freshly ground black pepper

mixed herbs, chopped parsley or celery salt, to taste

Heat the oven to 180°C/350°F/gas 4. Grease a 825 ml/1½ pt oven-proof dish.

Drain the lentils. Put them in a saucepan with 285 ml/½ pt water and bring to the boil. Cover the pan, reduce the heat to low and simmer, stirring occasionally, until the lentils are soft and the water is absorbed. Add more water if necessary.

Meanwhile, in a frying pan, fry the onion in the margarine over low heat for about 10 minutes or until soft but not brown. Add the tomatoes and cook for 5 minutes. Mash the lentils, add the cornflakes (reserving a few for the top), the onion mixture and the remaining ingredients. Adjust seasoning. Turn into the pie dish. Sprinkle with the reserved cornflakes and a little more grated cheese if liked. Bake for 30 minutes.

VEGETARIAN PILAFF

Each serving: 430 Cals/1810 kJ, 8 g fibre

1 tbsp olive oil
225 g/8 oz brown rice
4 celery stalks, sliced
3 medium onions, sliced
2 cloves garlic
½ tsp turmeric
60 g/2 oz dried fruit, e.g. currants or sultanas
115 g/4 oz mushrooms, roughly chopped
115 g/4 oz red or green peppers, chopped
1½ tsp gluten-free yeast extract, e.g. Marmite
1 tbsp lemon juice
freshly ground black pepper
115 g/4 oz salted peanuts
cress to garnish

Heat the oil in a saucepan and fry the rice gently until transparent. Add the celery, onions, garlic and turmeric. Stir and fry for a few more minutes. Add 550 ml/1 pt water, the dried fruit, mushrooms and peppers. Bring to the boil, stir, cover and simmer until the rice is tender and the water is absorbed. Stir in the yeast extract, lemon juice, freshly ground black pepper and nuts. Turn into a warmed serving dish and garnish with cress just before serving.

VEGETABLE CURRY

Each serving: 150 Cals/630 kJ, 8 g fibre

1 tbsp olive oil
1 medium onion, sliced
½ tsp ground ginger
1½ tsp turmeric
¼–1 tsp chilli powder, according to how hot you like curry
½ tsp ground coriander
2 tsp salt
freshly ground black pepper
400 g/14 oz tin tomatoes
1 apple, cored and sliced
handful mixed dried fruit (eg, currants and sultanas)

1 medium potato, sliced
a selection of vegetables, e.g.:
   340 g/12 oz runner beans, stringed and sliced
   2 medium carrots, sliced
   170 g/6 oz cauliflower, separated into small florets
   115 g/4 oz courgettes, sliced
   115 g/4 oz marrow, seeds removed and cut into cubes
1 tbsp lemon juice
1½ tsp gluten-free garam masala

Heat the oil in a large saucepan. Gently fry the onion and ginger for about 10 minutes. Stir in the turmeric, chilli, coriander, salt and freshly ground black pepper. Add the tomatoes with their juice, the apple, dried fruit and remaining vegetables. Bring to the boil, cover and simmer until all the vegetables are tender. Stir in the lemon juice and garam masala. Continue to simmer with the lid off so that the sauce can thicken a little.

Serve with plain boiled rice and Cucumber raita (page 62).

SPAGHETTI CHEESE IN TOMATO SAUCE

Each serving: 580 Cals/2430 kJ, 4 g fibre

115 g/4 oz gluten-free spaghetti
60 g/2 oz Cheddar cheese, grated
1 quantity Fresh tomato sauce (page 148)
2 tbsp gluten-free breadcrumbs
1 tsp dried mixed herbs
15 g/½ oz margarine
30 g/1 oz Parmesan cheese, grated

Heat the oven to 190°C/375°F/gas 5. Grease a deep pie dish.

Cook the pasta according to the manufacturer's instructions. Drain and rinse in cold water. Place half the pasta in the pie dish. Sprinkle with the Cheddar cheese. Cover with the rest of the pasta and pour the sauce over. Sprinkle with the breadcrumbs mixed with the herbs. Dot with the margarine and sprinkle the Parmesan cheese on top. Bake uncovered for about 30 minutes or until the top is crisp and golden.

Freeze before the baking stage. Thaw before baking.

Pizza

Makes 6 slices
Each slice: 420 Cals/1760 kJ, 2 g fibre

1 recipe basic White scones mixture (page 94) using 225 g/8 oz
    gluten-free flour and omitting the sugar

Topping:

1 medium onion, chopped

1 tbsp olive oil

3 fresh (or tinned) tomatoes, skinned and chopped

pinch sugar

salt and freshly ground black pepper

½ tsp oregano

115 g/4 oz cheese, grated

60 g/2 oz mushrooms, sliced

Heat the oven to 200°C/400°F/gas 6.

Sauté the chopped onion in the oil for 7–10 minutes. Add the
tomatoes and cook for 5 minutes more. Add the sugar, salt, pepper
and oregano to taste. Set aside to cool.

Meanwhile, pat the scone mixture into an 18–20cm/7–8 in round.
Place on a greased ovenproof plate or baking tray.

When the topping is cold spread on top of the base. Put the cheese
on top and decorate with slices of mushroom. Put the pizza in the oven
and bake for 20 minutes. Reduce the heat to 190°C/375°F/gas 5 and
bake for a further 10–15 minutes. Freezes well.

For a change use Brown scones base (page 95).

Savoury flan

A flan base can be made using either the Shortcrust pastry recipe (page 114) or the basic Brown pastry recipe given here. Three fillings are given but other gluten-free fillings can be used.

Brown pastry flan base

Flan base: 710 Cals/2970 kJ, 9 g fibre

60 g/2 oz hard margarine or butter
115 g/4 oz Glutafin gluten-free fibre mix
2–3 tbsp cold water

Heat the oven to 200°C/400°F/gas 6.

Rub the fat into the Glutafin mix until the mixture resembles breadcrumbs. Add enough water to give a soft but not sticky dough. Turn on to a surface lightly dusted with Glutafin mix and knead until smooth. Roll out and use to line an 18-cm/7-in flan dish. Prick the base of the flan well. Line with foil and weight down with dried beans or rice. Bake for 10–15 minutes to set the pastry. Remove the foil and beans.

Flan fillings:

Courgettes and red pepper

Filling, for one flan: 730 Cals/3070 kJ, 1 g fibre

30 g/1 oz margarine
2 small courgettes, thinly sliced
1 small red pepper, thinly sliced
1 large clove garlic, crushed
salt and freshly ground black pepper
60 g/2 oz Edam cheese, grated
140 ml/5 fl oz milk
1 egg

Mushroom and cheese

Filling, for one flan: 590 Cals/2480 kJ, 3 g fibre

30 g/1 oz margarine
60–120 g/2–4 oz mushrooms, sliced
1 medium onion, thinly sliced
salt and freshly ground black pepper
60 g/2 oz Edam cheese, grated
140 ml/5 fl oz milk
1 egg

Heat the oven to 200°C/400°F/gas 6.

In a frying pan, melt the margarine and fry the prepared vegetables for about 10 minutes. Season. Turn into the half-baked flan case and sprinkle with the cheese. Slightly warm the milk in the frying pan and pour on to the beaten egg. Adjust seasoning. Pour this custard over the vegetables, place the flan in the centre of the oven and bake for about 15 minutes or until browned and firm. Serve hot or cold.

YORKSHIRE PUDDING

Makes 8 individual puddings
Each pudding: 100 Cals/420 kJ, 0 g fibre

115 g/4 oz self-raising gluten-free flour*
pinch salt
1 egg
285 ml/½ pt milk and water (half and half)
30 ml/1 fl oz olive oil

Heat the oven to 220°C/425°F/gas 7.

Place the flour and salt in a mixing bowl: make a well in the centre with a wooden spoon. Drop the egg and half the milk and water into it. Gradually work the flour into the egg and milk to form a smooth cream. Slowly add the rest of the milk and water and beat well. Heat the oil in 8–10 patty tins or in a 23 x 18-cm/9 x 7-in tin, in the oven. When the oil begins to smoke, pour in the batter. Bake in the top of the oven until well risen and brown (about 20 minutes for the small puddings or 45 minutes for the large pudding). Serve immediately.
*Tested with Juvela gluten-free mix

PANCAKES

Makes 4 small pancakes
Each pancake: 120 Cals/500 kJ, 0 g fibre

2 tbsp plain gluten-free flour
pinch salt
1 egg
6 tbsp milk
4 tsp olive oil

Sift the flour and salt together into a bowl. Make a well in the centre, drop in the egg and 1 tablespoon of the milk. Beat with a wooden spoon until smooth. Continue beating for 2–3 minutes. Beat in the rest of the milk. Leave to stand for at least 5 minutes. Alternatively, combine all the ingredients in a blender.

Heat the oil in a 15-cm/6-in heavy frying pan and when very hot pour it off into a cup. Remove the pan from the heat, stir the batter and pour in a quarter of it. Replace the pan on the heat and cook quickly. When the edges begin to curl, turn the pancake and cook the other side. Turn on to a hot plate and keep warm. Repeat with the rest of the batter, reheating the oil in the pan and tipping it out before cooking the next pancake.

Fillings
Sweet
Squeeze lemon juice on to each pancake, sprinkle with 2 teaspoons sugar and roll up.

Savoury
Fill each pancake with 2 tablespoonfuls of any hot savoury filling, e.g. vegetables in a thick cheese sauce or minced left-over meat or chicken in a mushroom sauce (see White sauce, page 147). Place the rolled-up pancakes in an ovenproof dish, cover with more sauce, sprinkle with grated cheese and reheat in the oven at 200°C/400°F/gas 6 for 15 minutes.

Breads and Teabreads

Gluten gives structure to bread and when gluten-free flour is used bread tends to be more crumbly and cake-like. In the past, although a few local bakeries made gluten-free bread, most people made their own by hand or used packaged gluten-free bread produced by large commercial bakeries. The advent of the bread-making machine for use at home has provided an excellent alternative. Some, if not all, manufacturers of bread-making machines provide recipes and support for gluten-free bread making. The results are excellent.

Or you may prefer to make your bread by hand: if so, there is a variety of gluten-free flours and bread mixes available. It is best to use the type of flour stated in the recipe (self-raising or plain). The raising agents used are yeast or gluten-free baking powder. Yeast can be bought fresh from bakers or health food stores or dry from chemists, grocers and supermarkets. Fresh yeast will keep for up to three days in a loosely tied polythene bag in a cool place, and up to a week in a refrigerator. It can be frozen: weigh out in 15 g/½ oz or 30 g/1 oz cubes and wrap individually in polythene with a date label. The storage time will be four to six weeks in a freezer. Dried yeast will keep for six months if stored in a tightly sealed tin in a cool place. An alternative is fast-action dried yeast, which can be added straight into the flour mix.

Fifteen grams/½ oz dried yeast is equivalent to 30 g/1 oz fresh yeast. Yeast mixtures rise best if the moisture is kept in. This may be done by covering the tin with a sheet of lightly greased polythene or slipping the tin into a lightly greased polythene bag during rising.

The time the dough takes to rise in the tin varies with the temperature – about 45 minutes in a warm place – a little over an hour at room temperature. Do not over-raise yeast mixtures or they will collapse on baking.

To test if bread is cooked, tip it out of the tin and tap the bottom of the loaf – it should sound hollow. Gluten-free bread goes stale quickly, and if you are making it in bulk, you should freeze it immediately after baking and cooling. Do not store bread in the refrigerator as this accelerates staling. Slice loaves before freezing so you can defrost just as much as you need. Put the loaf in a plastic bag and seal, excluding as much air as possible. Many people find that gluten-free bread is better toasted and you can toast straight from the freezer.

Gluten-free bread will keep well in a freezer for up to six months. Thaw at room temperature for three to four hours or in a refrigerator overnight. Refresh in a hot oven for 5 minutes. Stale bread can be toasted or made into breadcrumbs and stored in an airtight container.

See also Baking and breadmaking, page 44, and Which flour to use?, page 52.

GLUTEN-FREE BAKING POWDER

85 g/3 oz cornflour
100 g/3½ oz bicarbonate of soda
60 g/2 oz cream of tartar
60 g/2 oz tartaric acid (from the chemist)

Mix all the ingredients together and pass through a fine sieve two or three times. Store in an airtight container in a dry place.

WHITE BREAD

Makes 2 small loaves
Each loaf: 910 Cals/3820 kJ, 0 g fibre

430 ml/¾ pt milk and water (half and half)
2 tsp dried yeast or 30 g/1 oz fresh yeast
1 tsp granulated sugar
340 g/12 oz plain gluten-free flour
1 tsp salt
30 g/1 oz lard

Grease two 450-g/1-lb loaf tins. Warm the milk and water until just comfortable to the touch. Put one-third of the milk and water in a bowl, sprinkle the dried yeast on to it and add a pinch of sugar; or, cream the fresh yeast with a pinch of sugar and a little of the warm liquid. In either case, leave to stand in a warm place for about 10 minutes until frothy.

Sift the flour and the salt, add the rest of the sugar and rub in the fat. Make a well in the centre and add the yeast and sufficient liquid to make a stiff batter. Beat, adding more milk and water as it thickens until you have a smooth batter that drops heavily from the spoon, adding more water if necessary. Divide the batter between the two tins, cover with oiled polythene or a damp cloth, and set in a warm place for 20–30 minutes or until risen to the top of the tins.

Heat the oven to 220°C/425°F/gas 7. Stand the tins on a baking sheet and bake for about 30 minutes, until well risen, firm and a light brown. Cool for a few minutes in the tin and turn on to a wire rack.

Slice and freeze if not to be used at once.

To make one large loaf allow 40–50 minutes and reduce the temperature to 200°C/400°F/gas 6 for the last 10 minutes.

BROWN BREAD

Makes 1 small loaf
710 Cals/2970 kJ, 9 g fibre

250 g/½ packet Glutafin gluten-free fibre mix
5 g/½ sachet easy-blend dried yeast enclosed with mix
pinch salt
½ tbsp olive oil
225ml/8 fl oz hand hot water

Grease a 450-g/1-lb loaf tin.

Put all the ingredients into a bowl. Mix well, using an electric mixer, for approximately 2 minutes to give a smooth, thick batter. Spoon into the loaf tin, brush the top with a little extra olive oil and cover with oiled polythene. Leave to prove in a warm place until the batter is level with the top of the tin. Heat the oven to 220°C/425°F/gas 7. Bake for approximately 25 minutes until the top is golden brown and firm to the touch.

To make rolls, either divide the batter between six greased bap tins or reduce the amount of water used to 140 ml/5 fl oz to form a soft, kneadable dough. Shape as desired. Bake for 10–15 minutes.

SUN-DRIED TOMATO BREAD

Serves 10

Each serving: 100 Cals/410 kJ, 1 g fibre

250 g/9 oz Glutafin gluten-free mix

2 tsp dried yeast enclosed with mix

pinch salt

1 tbsp olive oil

200 ml/7 fl oz tepid water

25 g/1 oz sun-dried tomatoes, chopped

pinch dried basil

15 g/½ oz sun-dried tomatoes for topping, chopped extra fine

Place the mix, yeast and salt in a large mixing bowl and mix together. Add the oil and water and beat with an electric mixer for 2 minutes on slow speed. Scrape down and beat again for 2 minutes on medium speed to form a smooth batter. Stir in the chopped tomatoes and herbs. Spoon into a greased 1-kg/2-lb loaf tin, brush with a little extra oil and sprinkle with the extra finely chopped tomatoes. Cover with a greased polythene bag and leave the dough to rise in a warm place for approximately 30 minutes. The batter should almost reach the top of the tin. Heat the oven to 200°C/400°F/gas 6. Bake for about 25 minutes. Remove from the tin and cool on a wire tray.

Good sliced for sandwiches; goes well with soups.

HONEY AND SUNFLOWER SEED BREAD

Makes about 8 slices

Each slice: 150 Cals/630 kJ, 2 g fibre

250 g/9 oz Glutafin gluten-free bread mix

5 g/½ sachet of easy-blend dried yeast enclosed with mix

30 g/1 oz margarine

6 tbsp milk

6 tbsp water

1 tbsp clear honey

40 g/1½ oz sunflower seeds

oil for brushing

Combine the Glutafin mix and yeast in a bowl. Melt the margarine. Remove from the heat and add the milk, water and honey – the mixture should be just warm. Add the warm liquid to the dry ingredients and beat well until a smooth batter is formed. Stir in 30 g/1 oz of the sunflower seeds. Spoon into a greased 450-g/1-lb loaf tin. Brush with oil, cover with a polythene bag and leave to rise in a warm place until mixture reaches the top of the tin. Heat the oven to 200°C/400°F/gas 6. Sprinkle with the rest of the sunflower seeds and bake for 20–25 minutes. Remove from the tin and leave to cool on a rack.

To store
When cool, wrap the loaf in a polythene bag.

To reheat
Warm through for 5 minutes in a hot oven or a few seconds in a microwave.

WHITE SCONES

Makes 8

Each scone: 210 Cals/880 kJ, 1 g fibre

225 g/8 oz self-raising gluten-free flour
½ tsp salt
1 tsp gluten-free baking powder
60 g/2 oz hard margarine
60 g/2 oz granulated sugar
60 g/2 oz mixed dried fruit (optional)
approximately 140 ml/5 fl oz milk

Heat the oven to 200°C/400°F/gas 6. Grease a baking sheet.

Sift the flour, salt and baking powder into a bowl. Add the margarine cut into pieces and rub in until the mixture resembles breadcrumbs. Add the sugar and fruit if used and mix to a soft dough with the milk. Roll out on a board dusted with gluten-free flour to about 1 cm/½ in thick and cut into rounds with a plain cutter. Or divide into two, shape into rounds 1 cm/½ in thick and mark into four. Place on a baking sheet and bake 10–15 minutes for small scones or 20–25 minutes for the larger rounds. They should be well risen and browned. Cool on a wire tray.

Brown scones

Makes 8
710 Cals/2970 kJ, 9 g fibre

225 g/8 oz Glutafin gluten-free fibre mix
pinch salt
2 tsp gluten-free baking powder
60 g/2 oz margarine
30 g/1 oz caster sugar
1 egg, beaten with sufficient milk to make 140 ml/5 fl oz

Heat the oven to 220°C/425°F/gas 7. Put the Glutafin mix, salt and baking powder in a bowl and mix well together. Rub in the margarine and stir in the sugar. Add enough of the egg and milk to give a soft dough. Turn on to a surface lightly dusted with Glutafin mix and gently knead until smooth. Roll out to 1 cm/½ in thick and cut into 6.5 cm/2½ in rounds. Brush with any remaining egg and milk and bake for 10 minutes.

Alternatives

For cheese scones, omit sugar and add 60–85 g/2–3oz grated hard cheese.
For fruit scones, add 60–85 g/2–3 oz dried fruit with the sugar.
For pizza base, omit sugar.

Butter cob

Makes 2 loaves or 16 small rolls
Each roll: 160 Cals/670 kJ, 0 g fibre

450 g/1 lb plain gluten-free flour
pinch salt
2 tsp gluten-free baking powder
115 g/4 oz butter
½ tsp sugar
285 ml/½ pt milk (or more, as required)

Heat the oven to 200°C/400°F/gas 6. Dust a baking sheet with gluten-free flour.

Sift the flour, salt and baking powder into a large bowl, rub in the fat and add the sugar. Mix with sufficient milk to make a sticky dough. Knead lightly to bring it together. Form into two large cobs 2–4 cm/1–1½ in thick and mark the tops with a cross.

Bake the loaves for 20 minutes and then reduce the heat to 190°C/375°F/gas 5 for 10 minutes, covering with greaseproof paper if browning too quickly.

Alternatives

Make into 16 small rolls or a pizza base, using one-third of the amounts for an 18-cm/7-in pizza. Bake the rolls for 15 minutes at 200°C/400°F/gas 6.

CORN BREAD

Makes 16 slices
Each slice: 80 Cals/340 kJ, 0 g fibre

115 g/4 oz cornmeal
115 g/4 oz plain gluten-free flour
1 tsp salt
3 tsp gluten-free baking powder
1 tbsp brown sugar
1 egg
200 ml/7 fl oz milk
60 g/2 oz butter, melted

Heat the oven to 220°C/425°F/gas 7. Grease a 20-cm/8-in square tin.

Sift the cornmeal, flour, salt and baking powder into a bowl. Stir in the sugar. Beat the egg lightly and add the milk and melted butter. Stir into the dry ingredients, mixing well. Pour the mixture into the tin and bake for 20–30 minutes, until lightly browned. Cool in the tin for 5 minutes and remove to a cooling rack.

BANANA BRAN BREAD

Makes 16 slices
Each slice: 160 Cals/670 kJ, 4 g fibre

115 g/4 oz soft margarine
115 g/4 oz soft brown sugar
1 egg
2 large ripe bananas
225 g/8 oz plain gluten-free flour
1 tsp gluten-free baking powder
1 tsp gluten-free mixed spice
85 g/3 oz raisins
60 g/2 oz soya bran
milk to mix, as necessary

Heat the oven to 180°C/350°F/gas 4. Grease a 1-kg/2-lb loaf tin and line the bottom with greaseproof paper.

Cream the margarine and sugar until light. Beat the egg, mash the bananas and gradually add to the creamed mixture. Sift together the flour, baking powder and spice, and add the dried fruit, bran and sufficient milk to form a stiff dropping mixture. Spoon into the tin, level the mixture and bake in the centre of the oven for 1¼–1½ hours. Leave in the tin for 5 minutes, then remove to a cooling tray. Store in a polythene bag in a cool place. Freezes well.

This loaf can be served as a plain cake or sliced and buttered.

BRAN FRUIT LOAF

Makes 2 small loaves
Each slice: 60 Cals/250 kJ, 5 g fibre

400 g/14 oz mixed dried fruit
340 ml/12 fl oz cold tea
250 g/9 oz plain gluten-free flour
3 tsp gluten-free baking powder
¼ tsp gluten-free mixed spice
115 g/4 oz soya bran
70 g/2½ oz brown sugar
2 eggs, beaten

Heat the oven to 180°C/350°F/gas 4. Grease two 450-g/1-lb loaf tins well.

Soak the fruit in the tea for at least 30 minutes. Sift the flour, baking powder and mixed spice in a bowl. Mix in the soya bran and the sugar. Add the fruit, tea and eggs and beat together well. Divide the mixture between the two loaf tins and bake for 1 hour or until brown and firm. Leave in the tin for a few minutes and then turn out on to a cooling rack.

DATE AND WALNUT LOAF

Makes 16 slices
Each slice: 190 Cals/800 kJ, 1 g fibre

225 g/8 oz chopped dates
170 g/6 oz demerara sugar
85 g/3 oz margarine
grated rind 1 orange
2 tbsp orange juice
1 egg
225 g/8 oz plain gluten-free flour
1½ tsp gluten-free baking powder
1 tsp ground cinnamon
60 g/2 oz chopped walnuts

Heat the oven to 180°C/350°F/gas 4. Grease a 1-kg/2-lb loaf tin and line the bottom with greased greaseproof paper.

Simmer the dates with 140 ml/5 fl oz water in a covered pan for 15 minutes or until soft. The water should all be absorbed by the time the dates are cooked; if it tends to dry out, add more. Stir in the sugar and margarine and remove the pan from the heat. Add the grated orange rind and juice and beat in the egg. Sift the flour, baking powder and cinnamon together and add to the mixture. Add the walnuts. Mix well and spoon into the prepared tin. Bake for 70–80 minutes, until a skewer comes out clean. Cool in the tin for 5 minutes, then remove to a wire rack. Store wrapped in foil in a cool place.

Cheese and chive loaf

Makes about 12 slices
Each slice: 170 Cals/725 kJ, 2.5 g fibre

225 g/8 oz Glutafin gluten-free white mix
225 g/8 oz Glutafin gluten-free fibre mix
10 g/1 sachet of easy-blend dried yeast enclosed with mix
½ tsp salt
½ tsp gluten-free mustard (optional)
360 ml/13 fl oz tepid water
1 tbsp olive oil
115 g/4 oz grated cheese
2 tsp fresh chives, chopped or 1 tsp dried chives

Oil a 1-kg/2-lb loaf tin.

Put all the ingredients except 30 g/1 oz of the cheese in a large bowl. Mix well, using an electric mixer, for approximately 2 minutes to give a soft thick batter. Or beat with a wooden spoon for 5 minutes to obtain a smooth batter. Spoon into the loaf tin and sprinkle with the rest of the cheese. Cover with an oiled polythene bag and leave to rise in a warm place until doubled in size and the mixture is level with the top of the tin. Heat the oven to 220°C/425°F/gas 7. Bake for approximately 20 minutes until golden brown in colour. Remove from the tin and leave to cool. To store, wrap in a polythene bag. To reheat, warm through for 5 minutes in a hot oven or a few seconds in a microwave.

Canadian muffins

Makes 6
Each muffin: 130 Cals/550 kJ, 0 g fibre

1 egg
60 ml/2 fl oz milk
1 tbsp melted butter
115 g/4 oz plain gluten-free flour
pinch salt
1½ tsp gluten-free baking powder
15 g/½ oz granulated sugar

Heat the oven to 200°C/400°F/gas 6. Grease six muffin tins or patty tins.

Beat the egg and milk in a bowl. Add the melted butter and stir well. Sift the gluten-free flour, salt and gluten-free baking powder together and stir in the sugar. Add the egg mixture to the dry ingredients, stirring only just enough to mix. *Do not beat* and do not mix until smooth; the batter should be coarse and stiff. Place 2 heaped teaspoonfuls in each tin. Bake for 20 minutes or until well risen and brown.

Best served warm immediately after cooking. If the muffins are left to go cold, they can be rewarmed by being wrapped loosely in aluminium foil and heated in a hot oven (230°C/450°F/gas 8) for 5 minutes.

For savoury or sweet muffins add the following:
60 g/2 oz crisp cooked bacon pieces (omit sugar)
60 g/2 oz grated cheese (omit sugar)
60 g/2 oz chopped nuts
60 g/2 oz any dried fruit

These should be mixed with the dry ingredients.

RUSSIAN PANCAKES (BLINI)

Makes 20
Each pancake: 40 Cals/170 kJ, 0 g fibre

115 g/4 oz buckwheat flour
45 g/1½ oz Glutafin gluten-free fibre mix
1 tsp gluten-free baking powder
½ tsp bicarbonate of soda
¼ tsp salt
1 tsp sugar
340 ml/12 fl oz buttermilk or milk soured with 1 tsp vinegar

Grease a griddle or heavy frying pan. Sift the buckwheat flour into a bowl with the bread mix, baking powder, bicarbonate of soda and salt – tip in any grain that remains in the sieve. Add the sugar. Add the buttermilk or soured milk to the dry ingredients, stirring to combine. Do not beat. This forms a very thin batter. Leave to stand for a few minutes.

Warm the griddle on a medium heat. Drop tablespoons of the batter carefully on to the griddle, leaving room for them to spread.

They will form about 7 cm/3 in pancakes. Cook for 2–3 minutes until bubbles appear on the surface. They will lift easily with a palette knife. Turn and cook for a further 2–3 minutes. Regrease the griddle or pan between additions as necessary. Pile onto a dish and keep warm. Serve at once.

These go well with breakfast dishes such as bacon, sausages and scrambled eggs. They are equally good with honey, maple syrup or jam.

Welsh griddle cakes

Makes 12

Each cake: 150 Cals/630 kJ, 1 g fibre

olive oil to grease the griddle
225 g/8 oz plain gluten-free flour
pinch salt
1½ tsp gluten-free baking powder
¼ tsp grated nutmeg or gluten-free mixed spice (optional)
85 g/3 oz hard margarine
60 g/2 oz granulated sugar
60 g/2 oz currants
1 egg
a little milk to mix
caster sugar to dust

Grease and heat a griddle or heavy frying pan to a moderate heat. Sift the gluten-free flour, salt and gluten-free baking powder and mixed spice, if using, into a bowl. Rub in the fat and add the sugar and currants. Beat the egg, add about a tablespoonful of milk, pour on to the dry mixture and bring together. Work into a stiff paste, adding more milk if necessary. Turn out on to a board dusted with gluten-free flour and pat or roll into a circle, not less than 5 mm/¼ in thick. Cut into triangles or rounds with a cutter. Lift with a palette knife on to the hot griddle. Cook each side for 4–5 minutes or until set, adjusting the heat as necessary. When cooked lift on to a piece of greaseproof paper and dust with sugar on both sides.

Serve immediately, or buttered when cold.

Puddings

As well as the recipes in this section, sago and tapioca are gluten-free, and fruit is an easy and healthy way to end a meal. Ready-made pie fillings, dessert mixes and ice-creams may contain gluten (see also the table on page 39).

Cold puddings

MUESLI

Each serving (dry): 180 Cals/760 kJ, 7 g fibre

60 g/2 oz gluten-free rolled oats

2 tbsp soya bran

2 tbsp sunflower seeds

30 g/1 oz chopped walnuts

30 g/1 oz stoned dates

30 g/1 oz raisins

Mix all the ingredients together. They may be combined in a large quantity and stored in a screw-top jar. Grated eating apple or fresh or stewed fruit in season may be added, and the muesli sweetened with honey or brown sugar. Muesli can be eaten alone or with milk or gluten-free yoghurt. For those who cannot tolerate oats, substitute another tablespoon of soya bran and more sunflower seeds and add some desiccated coconut.

PINEAPPLE CHEESECAKE

Makes 12 slices
Each slice: 210 Cals/880 kJ, 0 g fibre

Base:

9 gluten-free digestive biscuits
60 g/2 oz margarine
30 g/1 oz demerara sugar
a little ground cinnamon (optional)

Top:

15 g/½ oz powdered gelatin
115 ml/4 fl oz pineapple juice
170 g/6 oz pineapple pieces
2 eggs, separated
85 g/3 oz caster sugar
225 g/8 oz sieved cottage cheese
140 ml/5 fl oz soured or double cream
angelica to decorate

Grease an 18–20cm/7–8 in loose-bottomed cake tin.

To make the base, crush the biscuits. Melt the margarine and mix with the sugar, cinnamon and biscuit crumbs. Press the mixture on to the base of the tin and leave in a cool place to set.

Meanwhile, put the gelatin and the pineapple juice in a cup. Stand the cup in a pan of barely simmering water and stir until the gelatin has dissolved. Leave to cool. Cut up the pineapple into small pieces, reserving a few for decoration. In a mixing bowl, beat the egg yolks and sugar until light and thick. Add the dissolved gelatin, the cheese and the soured or double cream. Beat again and stir in the pineapple pieces. Lastly, when it is on the point of setting, fold in the stiffly beaten egg whites. Pour on to the prepared base and leave to set in the refrigerator (about 2–3 hours). Remove from the tin and slide the cake on to a serving plate. Decorate with pieces of pineapple and angelica.

Alternatives

Lemon or orange cheesecake: use the grated rind and juice of two lemons or two oranges in place of the pineapple pieces and the pineapple juice.

Strawberries or raspberries (115 g/4 oz) can be used as a topping for a lemon cheesecake.

Sponge flan base

Makes 8 slices
Each slice: 80 Cals/340 kJ, 0 g fibre

2 eggs
60 g/2 oz caster sugar
70 g/2½ oz plain gluten-free flour

Heat the oven to 200°C/400°F/gas 6. Grease a sponge flan tin 20 cm/8 in in diameter and place on a baking sheet.

Whisk the eggs and sugar together until thick and light. The mixture must leave a trail from the whisk which remains for a few seconds. Sift the flour on to the mixture and fold in very lightly with a metal spoon. Finally, fold in 1 tablespoonful of boiling water. Do not mix or beat any further. Pour the batter into the tin and bake for 15 minutes. The sponge should be firm, golden brown and springy to the touch. Leave to cool in the tin for at least 5 minutes. Ease out carefully and cool on a wire rack with the top side down.

Suggested fillings

When cold, fill with seasonal fresh fruit such as strawberries or raspberries, or any drained tinned fruit. If using fresh fruit, stew a few berries in about 140 ml/5 fl oz of water to extract the flavour. Drain the juice and measure it. Take 200 ml/7 fl oz of juice; blend a tablespoonful of cornflour with a little of the juice and bring the rest to the boil. Pour on to the cornflour, return to the pan and boil for 5 minutes, until it coats the back of a spoon. Sweeten to taste. Pour over the flan. If using tinned fruit, use the juice in the same way, but it may not need any extra sugar.

LEMON MERINGUE PIE

Serves 6
Each serving: 330 Cals/1390 kJ, 0 g fibre

Pastry base:
115 g/4 oz gluten-free flour
pinch salt
60 g/2 oz hard margarine
1 egg, beaten
Filling:
30 g/1 oz cornflour
grated rind and juice 2 lemons
115 g/4 oz granulated sugar
2 eggs, separated

Heat the oven to 200°C/400°F/gas 6.

Make the pastry (see Shortcrust pastry, page 114), roll it out on a surface dusted with gluten-free flour and line a flan tin or deep pie plate 18 cm/7 in in diameter. Prick the pastry all over with a fork. Line with foil and weight down the foil with dried beans or rice. Bake the pastry case for 15 minutes. Remove the foil and beans or rice and bake for a further 5 minutes to brown. Remove the pastry case from the oven and reduce the temperature to 150°C/300°F/gas 2.

Meanwhile prepare the filling. Blend the cornflour, lemon rind and juice, and 140 ml/5 fl oz water in a saucepan. Bring to the boil, stirring all the time, then simmer for a few minutes. Remove from the heat and add all but 2 tablespoonfuls of the sugar. Beat the egg yolks into the mixture. Pour into the pastry case. Whip the egg whites stiffly and fold in the 2 tablespoonfuls of sugar. Pile the meringue on top of the pie, covering the filling completely. Place in the cool oven for 15–20 minutes to set and brown lightly. Serve warm or cold. Do not freeze.

Fruit sorbet

Each serving: 150 Cals/630 kJ, 8 g fibre

450 g/1 lb soft fruit
115 g/4 oz granulated sugar
285 ml/½ pt water
1 tsp gelatin
2 egg whites

Turn the refrigerator to the lowest setting or turn on the fast-freeze section of the freezer.

Purée the fruit and sieve if necessary to remove seeds. In a saucepan, dissolve the sugar in the water and bring to the boil. Boil rapidly for 5 minutes and set aside to go cold. Sprinkle the gelatin over a little water in a pan and when soaked heat gently to dissolve. Then mix together the syrup, purée and gelatin and put into a suitable container. Freeze until just mushy, about 30 minutes. Stir to remove ice crystals around the edges. Whisk the egg whites until stiff and fold into the purée. Return to the freezer for at least 2 hours. To serve allow to defrost for 10–15 minutes – the exact time will depend on the temperature of your freezer and the fruit used.

Danish biscuits (page 122) go well with this.

Raspberry mousse

Each serving: 240 Cals/1010 kJ, 5 g fibre

425 g/15 oz tin raspberries
130 g/1 packet raspberry jelly (to make 550 ml/1 pt)
170 g/6 oz tin evaporated milk
1 tsp lemon juice

Strain the raspberries and measure the juice. Make up to 285 ml/½ pt with water. Place the juice in a pan, add the jelly and warm, stirring until it is dissolved. Do not allow to boil. Leave to cool and refrigerate until it is beginning to set. Purée the raspberries. Place the evaporated milk and lemon juice in a bowl and whisk until the mixture is very thick and will hold soft peaks. Fold in the raspberry purée and the jelly. Pour into a serving dish and leave to set, preferably in a refrigerator.

Other fruit and a correspondingly flavoured jelly can be used.

Fruit and nut iced cake

Serves 12

Each serving: 170 Cals/710 kJ, 1 g fibre

115 g/4 oz mixed dried fruit

60 g/2 oz maraschino cherries or washed glacé cherries, quartered

2 tbsp sherry

200 ml/7 fl oz milk

1 tsp powdered gelatin

1 tsp powdered instant coffee

1 tsp gluten-free cocoa

60 g/2 oz chopped walnuts

60 g/2 oz caster sugar (to taste)

a few drops vanilla essence

285 ml/½ pt whipping cream

chopped nuts and cherries

Turn the refrigerator to the lowest setting or switch on the fast-freeze section of the freezer.

Mix the fruits and the sherry and leave to stand for about 30 minutes. Warm the milk and dissolve the gelatin in it. Add the coffee and cocoa. Remove from the heat and cool in a large bowl. When cold add the soaked fruit and sherry, nuts, sugar and vanilla essence. Whip the cream until it forms soft peaks, fold into the fruit mixture and turn into a bowl. Freeze for about 1 hour. Take out of the freezer and mix well with a fork to distribute the fruit evenly. Re-freeze until required.

Remove from freezer 30 minutes before serving. Dip the bowl into hot water for a second and turn on to a serving dish. Sprinkle with the nuts and cherries.

Dutch fruit salad

Each serving: 180 Cals/760 kJ, 4 g fibre

225 g/8 oz tin pineapple pieces

60 g/2 oz sugar (optional)

rind 1 lemon

juice ½ lemon

340 g/12 oz fresh fruit, e.g. apples, plums, oranges, melon, grapes or soft fruit

1–2 tbsp kirsch
chopped preserved ginger (optional)

Drain the pineapple, saving the juice. Make the juice up to 285 ml/½ pt with water or orange juice. Place in a small saucepan with the sugar. Add the lemon rind and juice. Heat gently, stirring to dissolve the sugar. Bring to the boil and simmer for 5 minutes. Leave to infuse for 20 minutes. Meanwhile prepare the fruits, cutting them into suitably sized pieces (if using bananas, slice into the salad just before serving). Pour the cooled syrup over the fruit. Stir in the kirsch, and pieces of ginger, if using. Chill in the refrigerator.

SIMPLE ICE-CREAM

Each serving: 340 Cals/1430 kJ, 0 g fibre

285 ml/½ pt milk
2 tbsp gluten-free custard powder
115 g/4 oz caster sugar
285 ml/½ pt double cream, well chilled, or 400 g/14 oz tin
  evaporated milk, well chilled
a few drops vanilla essence (optional)

Turn the refrigerator to its lowest setting or switch on the fast-freeze section of the freezer.

Make a custard with the milk and custard powder as directed on the packet. Add the sugar. Set aside to cool. Whip the cream or evaporated milk until very thick. Add the cold custard and mix well. Flavour if desired with vanilla essence. Pour into freezing trays and freeze until just set round the sides. Return to a bowl and whisk. Replace in the freezing trays and freeze until hard. Store in the freezer. Remove from the freezer 30 minutes before required and keep in the refrigerator until served.

May be flavoured by adding gluten-free instant coffee or other gluten-free flavourings to the milk during the making of the custard.

Hot puddings

BAKED CUSTARD

Each serving: 170 Cals/710 kJ, 0 g fibre

2 eggs
30 g/1 oz granulated sugar
550 ml/1 pt milk
a few drops vanilla essence (optional)
grated nutmeg

Heat the oven to 170°C/325°F/gas 3. Grease a 825-ml/1½-pt pie dish.

Beat the eggs lightly with the sugar. Warm the milk to blood heat and pour on to the eggs and sugar. Mix well, adding vanilla essence if using. Pour the custard into the pie dish. Grate a little nutmeg on top. Place the pie dish in a tin of water in the oven; the water should come about halfway up the sides of the pie dish – this prevents the custard curdling. Bake for 1 hour or until the custard sets. Serve warm or cold.

Baked apples go well with this and can be baked at the same time.

FRUIT CRUMBLE

Serves 6
Each serving: 360 Cals/1510 kJ, 6 g fibre

450 g/1 lb fresh fruit, e.g. plums, cooking apples, gooseberries or rhubarb
115 g/4 oz brown sugar, according to taste; some fruits need more than others
Topping:
140 g/5 oz gluten-free flour
30 g/1 oz soya bran
85 g/3 oz hard margarine
60 g/2 oz walnuts or toasted hazelnuts, finely chopped (optional)
30 g/1 oz demerara sugar

Heat the oven to 180°C/350°F/gas 4. Grease a 825-ml/1½-pt pie dish.

Prepare the fruit, mix with the brown sugar and place in the pie dish. Mix the gluten-free flour and soya bran and rub in the margarine until the mixture resembles fine breadcrumbs. Stir in the nuts, if using, and demerara sugar. Tip over the fruit and press down gently. Place in the centre of the oven. Bake for about 1 hour, until the fruit is tender. If the top browns too quickly, reduce the heat to 170°C/325°F/gas 3. Serve hot with gluten-free custard or cold with cream.

Alternatives
A little dried fruit or chopped ginger may be added to the raw fruit, and gluten-free mixed spice or cinnamon to the demerara sugar.

BROWN BETTY

Each serving: 440 Cals/1850 kJ, 4 g fibre

60 g/2 oz margarine
8 gluten-free digestive biscuits, crushed, or 85 g/3 oz dried gluten-free breadcrumbs
140 g/5 oz brown sugar
450 g/1 lb cooking apples
juice 1 lemon
1 tsp ground cinnamon
¼ tsp ground nutmeg
grated rind ½ lemon

Heat the oven to 180°C/350°F/gas 4. Grease a 1.5-l/2½-pt oven-proof dish.

Melt the margarine and add the bread or biscuit crumbs and 30 g/1 oz of the brown sugar. Mix well. Line the bottom of the dish with a third of this mixture. Peel, core and slice the apples very thinly and put in a bowl. Sprinkle with the lemon juice, and mix in the remaining brown sugar, spices, lemon rind and 2 tablespoonfuls of water. Stir well. Place half this mixture on top of the crumbs in the dish. Cover with a further third of the crumbs, repeat the fruit layer and top with the remainder of the crumbs. Press down lightly. Cover with greased greaseproof paper and bake in the centre of the oven for about 40 minutes or until the apples are nearly soft. Increase the heat to 200°C/400°F/gas 6, remove the greaseproof paper and cook for a further 15 minutes until the top is crisp and brown.

An alternative
Add a tablespoonful of mixed dried fruit to each layer of apples.

BAKED LEMON DELIGHT

Each serving: 280 Cals/1180 kJ, 0 g fibre

60 g/2 oz soft margarine
60 g/2 oz granulated sugar
2 eggs, separated
1 tbsp gluten-free flour
grated rind and juice 1 large lemon
285 ml/½ pt milk

Heat the oven to 180°C/350°F/gas 4. Grease a 825-ml/1½-pt pie or soufflé dish.

Cream the margarine and sugar together until very light. Beat in the egg yolks and then the flour, lemon rind and juice. Beat well. Mix in the milk carefully, do not worry if it curdles a little. Beat the egg whites until they just hold peaks and fold in carefully. Pour into the greased dish and bake for 45 minutes. It should be slightly risen and firm on top. Serve hot or cold.

ORANGE PUDDING

Each serving: 320 Cals/1340 kJ, 0 g fibre

60 g/2 oz soft margarine
60 g/2 oz caster sugar
1 egg
grated rind 1 orange
85 g/3 oz plain gluten-free flour
pinch salt
¼ tsp gluten-free baking powder
1–2 tbsp milk
3 tbsp orange marmalade (optional)

Grease a 550-ml/1-pt pudding basin. In a mixing bowl, cream the margarine and sugar until light. Beat in the egg and orange rind. Sift together the gluten-free flour, salt and gluten-free baking powder and fold into the creamed mixture. Add milk as required to form a soft dropping consistency. Spread the marmalade, if using, on to the bottom of the basin and spoon in the mixture. Cover first with greased greaseproof paper, and then with foil, folding and twisting it over the rim of the basin to keep out the steam. Place in a steamer or in a covered pan containing water halfway up the sides of the basin. Bring to the boil and steam for 50–60 minutes. Carefully add more boiling water as necessary.

CHRISTMAS PUDDING

Each serving: 270 Cals/1130 kJ, 3 g fibre

30 g/1 oz plain gluten-free flour
⅛ tsp salt
¼ tsp gluten-free mixed spice
⅛ tsp bicarbonate of soda
grated rind ½ lemon
60 g/2 oz cooking apple, grated
60 g/2 oz brown sugar
30 g/1 oz chopped almonds
60 g/2 oz sultanas
60 g/2 oz currants
30 g/1 oz raisins
30 g/1 oz chopped mixed peel
45 g/1½ oz gluten-free shredded suet
70 g/2½ oz gluten-free breadcrumbs
1 egg
3–4 tbsp milk

Grease a 450-g/1-lb pudding basin. Sift the flour, salt, mixed spice and bicarbonate of soda into a large mixing bowl. Add the lemon rind, apple, sugar, almonds, dried fruit, shredded suet and breadcrumbs. Mix well. Beat the egg with the milk. Gradually stir into the mixture, which should form a soft dropping consistency: if it is too stiff, add a little more milk. Spoon into the basin, cover with greased greaseproof paper and then with foil. Place in a steamer or in a covered pan containing water halfway up the sides of the basin. Bring to the boil and steam for 5 hours, topping up with boiling water as necessary. Allow to cool. Cover with new foil or a cloth and seal well.

When ready for use, steam for 1–1½ hours and serve.

This pudding improves with keeping and can be stored for up to a year. If it becomes dry, moisten with a little cider or milk before re-steaming.

BREAD AND BUTTER PUDDING

Each serving: 550 Cals/2310 kJ, 2 g fibre

60 g/2 oz butter or margarine
6 slices gluten-free bread
4 tbsp thick marmalade (optional)
1 medium cooking apple, grated or thinly sliced
85 g/3 oz brown sugar
60 g/2 oz raisins
1 tsp ground cinnamon (optional)
2 eggs
430 ml/¾ pt milk

Grease a 1.5-l/2½-pt pie dish.

Butter each slice of bread and spread with marmalade, if using. Make a layer of the bread and marmalade in the bottom of the dish. Cover with half the apple, half the sugar and half the raisins, and some cinnamon if using. Repeat once and end with a layer of bread and marmalade, buttered side down. Dot with a little more butter and a sprinkling of sugar. Beat the eggs and milk together and pour over. Press down and leave to stand at least 30 minutes. Heat the oven to 180°C/350°F/gas 4. Bake for about 45 minutes or until the custard is set and the top is crispy. Serve hot or cold.

OLD-FASHIONED RICE PUDDING

Each serving: 240 Cals/1010 kJ, 3 g fibre (bran included)

700 ml/1¼ pt milk
60 g/2 oz pudding rice
15 g/½ oz soya bran (optional)
45 g/1½ oz granulated sugar
2 pieces lemon rind
15 g/½ oz margarine
½ tsp grated nutmeg

Heat the oven to 170°C/325°F/gas 3. Grease a 825-ml/1½-pt pie dish.

Warm the milk. Put the rice, bran (if using), sugar, lemon rind and margarine in the dish and pour the milk over. Stir to dissolve the sugar. Add the nutmeg and stir again. Bake for 2–3 hours, stirring once or twice during the first hour, and then leave undisturbed for the remaining time.

Pastries, Biscuits and Small Cakes

Gluten-free pastry is very good. If it cracks when it is being rolled out it is because it is too dry. Always add a few teaspoonfuls more water than you think necessary. Do not roll out too thinly: it should be about 5 mm/¼ in thick or more. If you are not going to use the pastry immediately, wrap it in a plastic bag or foil to prevent it drying out, and store in a refrigerator or freezer.

See also Baking and breadmaking, page 44, and Which flour to use? page 52.

SHORTCRUST PASTRY

Sufficient for 12 small tarts or 1 x 18 cm/7 in single pie crust
115 g/4 oz pastry: 950 Cals/3990 kJ, 0 g fibre

115 g/4 oz plain gluten-free flour
pinch salt
30 g/1 oz white vegetable fat (from the refrigerator)
30 g/1 oz hard margarine
1 egg

Sift the flour and salt into a bowl. Cut the fats into the flour and then, using your fingertips, rub in lightly until the mixture resembles dry breadcrumbs. Beat the egg with 1 tablespoonful cold water. Sprinkle it over the crumb mixture and mix lightly. This should form a pliable but not sticky dough. If you are not using the pastry immediately, make a wetter dough as it tends to dry out on standing. To roll out, lightly dust a board and a rolling pin with gluten-free flour, place the dough on the board and roll firmly, lifting and flouring underneath to prevent sticking. Do not roll less than 5 mm/¼ in thick. Use as required, and bake in an oven preheated to 200°C/400°F/gas 6.

NB There is no need to grease tins or dishes when using shortcrust pastry. It will not stick if you use at least half the quantity of fat to flour. Prick well before filling to prevent the pastry rising. You will need pastry made with 170 g/6 oz flour for a top and bottom crust tart 18 cm/7 in in diameter.

RICH SWEETCRUST PASTRY

Sufficient for 24 small tarts or 2 x 18 cm/7 in single pie crusts
225 g/8 oz pastry: 1930 Cals/8110 kJ, 0 g fibre

225 g/8 oz plain gluten-free flour
pinch salt
115 g/4 oz butter or hard margarine (from the refrigerator)
60 g/2 oz caster sugar
1 egg
1–2 tsp lemon juice

There is no need to grease the tins to be used.

Sift the flour and salt into a bowl. Cut the fat into small pieces and rub into the flour until the mixture resembles fine breadcrumbs. Stir in the sugar. Beat the egg with the lemon juice and sprinkle over the crumb mixture. Bring together gently and knead into a ball. Add a few drops of water if the pastry is too dry. It should form a soft pliable dough. Wrap the pastry in foil and chill for 30 minutes in the refrigerator. Do not roll out less than 5 mm/¼ in thick. Use as required, and bake in an oven preheated to 200°C/400°F/gas 6.

ALMOND FRUIT PASTRIES

Makes 6 wedges
Each wedge: 220 Cals/920 kJ, 2 g fibre

60 g/2 oz soft margarine
60 g/2 oz ground rice
60 g/2 oz plain gluten-free flour
1 large eating apple, unpeeled
60 g/2 oz plus a little extra soft brown sugar
30 g/1 oz ground almonds
flaked almonds to decorate

Heat the oven to 220°C/425°F/gas 7. Grease an ovenproof plate or tin 20 cm/8 in in diameter.

Blend the margarine, ground rice and flour together with a fork. Grate half the apple and mix it in with 60 g/2 oz of the sugar and the ground almonds. Knead into a ball. Press out on the plate. Thinly slice the rest of the apple and arrange in circles on the pastry, working towards the centre. Sprinkle with a little more sugar and decorate with the flaked almonds. Bake for 20 minutes, or until browned. Cut into wedges and serve warm or cold.

For a change, mix some cinnamon with the brown sugar sprinkled on the top.

WELSH CHEESE CAKES

Makes 12

Each cake: 230 Cals/970 kJ, 0 g fibre

½ quantity Rich sweetcrust pastry (page 115)

Filling:

raspberry jam

45 g/1½ oz soft margarine

45 g/1½ oz caster sugar

1 egg

30 g/1 oz plain gluten-free flour

60 g/2 oz ground rice

½ tsp gluten-free baking powder

a few drops vanilla essence

icing sugar

Heat the oven to 200°C/400°F/gas 6.

Roll and cut out the pastry into 6-cm/2½-in circles. Line 12 patty tins with the pastry and place a small teaspoonful of jam in each. In a bowl, cream the margarine and sugar until very light and beat in the egg. Sift together the flour, ground rice and baking powder. Fold into the creamed mixture with the vanilla essence. Divide equally between the 12 tarts. Bake for 15 minutes, then reduce the heat to 190°C/375°F/gas 5 for a further 5 minutes. Cool on a wire tray. Dust with icing sugar to serve.

PROFITEROLES OR CHOCOLATE ÉCLAIRS

Makes 15 éclairs or puffs
Each: 140 Cals/590 kJ, 0 g fibre

85 g/3 oz plain gluten-free flour
pinch salt
45 g/1½ oz hard margarine
2 eggs, medium (not larger)
140 ml/5 fl oz double or whipping cream, whipped until stiff
Chocolate glacé icing:
2 tsp gluten-free cocoa
170 g/6 oz icing sugar
Chocolate sauce:
45 g/1½ oz plain gluten-free cooking chocolate, broken into pieces
1 tsp cornflour
pinch salt
60 g/2 oz granulated sugar
a few drops vanilla essence
15 g/½ oz margarine

Heat the oven to 220°C/425°F/gas 7. Grease a large baking sheet. Sift the flour and salt together. Put 140 ml/5 fl oz water and the margarine in a small saucepan over heat. When the margarine has melted, bring to the boil. Tip in the flour all at once, remove the pan from the heat and beat until smooth. Beat one egg in until the mixture is smooth and glossy. Repeat with the second egg. It should form a stiff paste. For profiteroles, place teaspoonfuls on the baking sheet. For éclairs, pipe 7-cm/3-in lengths, using a 2-cm/1-in nozzle. Bake for 25–30 minutes in the middle of the oven. Do not open the door for at least 25 minutes. When the buns are well risen, browned and crisp remove from the oven. Cut a slit in each to allow the steam to escape and leave to cool on a wire rack. When cold fill with whipped cream. Cover with chocolate glacé icing (see below). Alternatively, the filled buns may be piled on a dish and chocolate sauce poured over them.

To make the icing

Dissolve the cocoa in a little warm water (1–2 tablespoonfuls) and gradually add to the icing sugar. The icing should be thick enough to coat the back of a spoon: if needed add water or sugar to adjust. Use at once.

To make the chocolate sauce

Add 115 ml/4 fl oz water to the chocolate in a small saucepan and melt over a low heat. Mix the cornflour and salt with a little water to make a smooth cream. Bring 85 ml/3 fl oz water to the boil and pour on to the blended cornflour, stirring. Return to the pan and bring back to the boil, stirring continuously. Add the chocolate and the sugar and cook for 4–5 minutes, stirring and beating. Finally, stir in the vanilla essence and the margarine, leave to cool and pour over the buns.

APPLE CINNAMON SHORTCAKE

Makes 12 pieces
Each piece: 150 Cals/630 kJ, 2 g fibre

140 g/45 oz plain gluten-free flour
1 tsp gluten-free baking powder
½ tsp cinnamon
30 g/1 oz soya bran
85 g/3 oz hard margarine
85 g/3 oz plus 1 tbsp caster sugar
1 egg, beaten
170 g/6 oz cooking apple, peeled, cored and thinly sliced

Heat the oven to 180°C/350°F/gas 4. Grease an 18-cm/7-in square or a 20-cm/8-in round tin and line with greaseproof paper. Sift the flour, baking powder and cinnamon together into a bowl. Mix in the bran, and rub in the margarine. Stir in 85 g/3 oz of the caster sugar. Work most of the egg into the mixture and knead until smooth, adding more egg if the pastry is too dry to roll out. Divide the pastry in half and roll out one half to fit the tin. Line the base of the tin with the pastry. Place a layer of apple over the top and press down. Roll out the other half of the pastry and place over the apple. Press down well and brush with a little milk. Mark with a fork and sprinkle with the extra tablespoon of sugar. Bake for 30–40 minutes or until lightly browned. Leave to cool in the tin. Lift out, peel off the paper and cut the shortcake into pieces. Will keep for several days, wrapped, in a refrigerator.

An alternative

Substitute ½ teaspoonful ground ginger for the cinnamon and spread a thick layer of ginger marmalade in place of the apple.

MINCE PIES

Makes 12
Each pie: 230 Cals/970 kJ, 0 g fibre

1 quantity Rich sweetcrust pastry (page 115)
340 g/12 oz gluten-free mincemeat
egg white or milk to glaze
icing sugar

Heat the oven to 200°C/400°F/gas 6.

Roll out the pastry, cut out 12 circles using a 6-cm/2½-in pastry cutter. Line 12 patty tins with the pastry. Cut the tops using a cutter one size smaller. Fill with the gluten-free mincemeat. Moisten the edges with water and cover with the tops, pressing the edges well down to seal. Make a slit in each top to let out the steam. Brush the tops with egg white or milk. Bake for 15–20 minutes or until golden brown. Cool on a wire rack and dust with icing sugar before serving.

SHORTBREAD

Makes 15 fingers
Each finger: 110 Cals/460 kJ, 0 g fibre

140 g/5 oz plain gluten-free flour
30 g/1 oz ground rice
60 g/2 oz granulated sugar plus a little for dusting
115 g/4 oz butter (not straight from the refrigerator, but not soft)

Heat the oven to 180°C/350°F/gas 4.

Mix the flour and ground rice in a large bowl and stir in the sugar. Place the butter in one piece in the bowl and work in with one hand, kneading until the mixture binds together and becomes smooth. Turn on to a board dusted with gluten-free flour and shape into a rectangle. Roll out to a strip 30 x 7 cm/12 x 3 in and about 1 cm/½ in thick. Nip the edges between thumb and forefinger as you go along to form a pattern. Prick well and dust with a little granulated sugar. Cut into fingers 1.5–2 cm/¾–1 in wide. Use a palette knife to place well apart on an ungreased baking sheet and bake in the middle of the oven for 20–30 minutes or until pale golden. Cool on the baking sheet. Store in an airtight tin when cold.

Basic biscuit mixture

Makes 36 biscuits
Each biscuit: 70 Cals/290 kJ, 1 g fibre

170 g/6 oz gluten-free flour
60 g/2 oz soya bran
115 g/4 oz soft margarine
170 g/6 oz caster sugar
1 egg
milk to mix, as necessary
Any of the following may be added to the mixture:
30–60 g/1–2 oz chopped nuts, candied peel, ginger pieces,
    chopped glacé cherries, grated orange or lemon rind, or gluten-
    free chocolate chips

Heat the oven to 190°C/375°F/gas 5. Grease two or three baking sheets.

Sift the flour into a bowl and add the other ingredients. Work together with a wooden spoon and then knead lightly to form a ball. Add a little milk if the dough will not hold together. Turn on to a board dusted with gluten-free flour and roll into a sausage not more than 30 cm/12 in long. Wrap it in greaseproof paper and refrigerate for 30 minutes. When firm cut into 5-mm/¼-in slices with a sharp knife and lift on to a baking sheet, leaving space for the slices to spread. Bake for 15–20 minutes, until well browned. Cool on a wire rack. Store in an airtight tin. If you wrap the dough in foil it freezes very well.

May be decorated with glacé icing and an almond or a cherry, or coated with melted gluten-free chocolate.

CHEESE BISCUITS

Makes 20
Each biscuit: 40 Cals/170 kJ, 0 g fibre

60 g/2 oz well-flavoured cheese, grated
85 g/3 oz plain gluten-free flour
dash cayenne pepper (optional)
½ tsp salt
60 g/2 oz hard margarine

Grease a baking sheet.

Mix the cheese, flour, cayenne pepper, if using, and salt in a bowl and rub the fat into them. Dust your hands with gluten-free flour and knead the mixture into a ball. Wrap the dough in clingfilm or greaseproof paper and refrigerate for 30 minutes. Heat the oven to 190°C/375°F/gas 5. Roll out on to a board dusted with gluten-free flour to 5 mm/¼ in thick. Prick well and cut into small biscuits. Put the biscuits on the baking sheet and bake for 10–15 minutes until pale gold – do not overcook or the cheese may become bitter. Cool on a wire rack and store in an airtight tin.

CRISP CRYSTAL BISCUITS

Makes 20
Each biscuit: 90 Cals/380 kJ, 2 g fibre

140 g/5 oz plain gluten-free flour
60 g/2 oz ground rice
85 g/3 oz caster sugar
60g/2oz soya bran
115 g/4 oz hard margarine
1 egg, separated
a little demerara sugar

Heat the oven to 180°C/350°F/gas 4. Grease two baking sheets.

Mix the flour, ground rice, sugar and bran in a bowl. Rub in the margarine until the mixture resembles fine breadcrumbs. Add the egg yolk and knead until smooth. Wrap the dough in greaseproof paper and refrigerate for 30 minutes. Roll out to 5 mm/¼ in thick. Use a 7-cm/3-in pastry cutter to cut out the biscuits. Brush with the lightly beaten egg white and sprinkle with demerara sugar. Bake for 15 minutes or until golden brown. Leave to cool a little and then remove to a cooling rack. Store in an airtight tin.

For variety add a little cinnamon to the sugar before sprinkling it over the biscuits.

DANISH BISCUITS

Makes 30

Each biscuit: 100 Cals/420 kJ, 2 g fibre

225 g/8 oz plain gluten-free flour
60 g/2 oz soya bran
170 g/6 oz slightly salted butter
115 g/4 oz granulated sugar
60 g/2 oz chopped almonds
2–3 drops almond essence
1 egg yolk, beaten
1 egg white, lightly beaten
a little granulated sugar
30 flaked almonds

Grease two baking sheets.

Mix the flour and bran together and lightly rub in the butter. It will be difficult so do not try to form 'fine breadcrumbs', just break it up. Add the sugar, almonds and essence and rub again to mix evenly. Bind together with the egg yolk. Turn on to a board lightly dusted with gluten-free flour. Form into a sausage and work into a smooth roll, not more than 30 cm/12 in long. Wrap in greaseproof paper and chill in the refrigerator until firm, at least 30 minutes. Heat the oven to 180°C/350°F/gas 4. Roll into walnut-sized balls, press flat and place well apart on the baking sheets. Brush with the lightly beaten egg white and sprinkle a little sugar on each. Decorate with an almond flake. Bake until golden brown, about 20 minutes. Leave on the trays for 5 minutes to set. Cool on a wire tray and store in an airtight tin.

New Zealand biscuits

Makes 30
Each biscuit: 90 Cals/380 kJ, 1 g fibre

140 g/5 oz hard margarine
1 tbsp golden syrup – measure with a warmed spoon
60 g/2 oz brown sugar
115 g/4 oz self-raising gluten-free flour
115 g/4 oz gluten-free rolled (porridge) oats
1 tsp ground ginger, or to taste
60 g/2 oz desiccated coconut
½ tsp bicarbonate of soda

Grease two baking sheets. Slowly melt the margarine, golden syrup and sugar in a large pan. Remove from the heat. Mix together the flour, oats, ginger and coconut. Dissolve the bicarbonate of soda in 1 tablespoonful hot water, add to the pan and then add the dry ingredients. Cool for 10–15 minutes or until the mixture becomes stiff. Heat the oven to 170°C/325°F/gas 3. Take walnut-sized pieces and pat into balls in your hands. Place on the prepared sheets and flatten slightly, leaving room for them to spread a little. Bake for 20–30 minutes, or until golden brown. Cool on a wire tray. The biscuits keep well stored in an airtight tin.

Plain oaten biscuits

Makes 24
Each biscuit: 70 Cals/290 kJ, 1 g fibre

85 g/3 oz gluten-free rolled (porridge) oats
115 g/4 oz medium gluten-free oatmeal
85 g/3 oz gluten-free flour
½ tsp salt
60 g/2 oz hard margarine
140 ml/5 fl oz (or as required) milk soured with 1 tsp vinegar

Heat the oven to 190°C/375°F/gas 5. Dust one or two baking sheets with gluten-free flour.

Mix the dry ingredients together in a large bowl. Rub in the margarine and mix with sufficient milk to make a soft sticky dough.

Place on a board lightly floured with gluten-free flour. Roll out to 5 mm/¼ in thick. Prick well. Cut into squares with a sharp knife or fluted potato chipper. Place on baking sheets and bake until lightly browned, 15–20 minutes. Remove to a cooling tray. Store in an airtight tin.

A plain biscuit to eat with cheese or jam. They keep well.

To make a sweet version of this biscuit add 60 g/2 oz demerara sugar.

OAT CRUNCHIES

Makes 20

Each biscuit: 90 Cals/380 kJ, 1 g fibre

115 g/4 oz hard margarine
130 g/4½ oz gluten-free rolled (porridge) oats
115 g/4 oz light brown sugar

Heat the oven to 190°C/375°F/gas 5. Grease a 28 x 18-cm /11 x 7-in baking tin and line it with greased greaseproof paper.

Gently melt the margarine; do not allow it to brown. Mix the oats and the sugar in a bowl. Pour the melted fat on to the mixture and mix well. Turn into the baking tin and press it down firmly with your hands. Bake in the centre of the oven for 15–20 minutes or until pale gold, turning the tin after 10 minutes to ensure even cooking. Cut into squares whilst still hot. Leave in the tin to cool. When cold store in an airtight tin.

FLAPJACKS

Makes 14
Each flapjack: 150 Cals/630 kJ, 1 g fibre

115 g/4 oz soft brown sugar
115 g/4 oz margarine
170 g/6 oz gluten-free rolled (porridge) oats
1 tbsp golden syrup – measure with a warmed spoon
¾ tsp ground ginger

Heat the oven to 150°C/300°F/gas 2. Grease a Swiss roll tin (28 x 18-cm/11 x 7-in).

Melt the sugar and margarine in a saucepan. Stir in the oats, syrup and ginger. Press the mixture evenly into the prepared tin. Bake for 40 minutes or until golden brown. Allow to cool slightly and mark into fingers with a sharp knife.

The flapjacks may be stored in an airtight tin for up to 1 week.

GINGER SNAPS

Makes 24 biscuits
Each biscuit: 90 Cals/380 kJ, 0 g fibre

225 g/8 oz Glutafin gluten-free white mix
2 tsp gluten-free baking powder
pinch salt
1 tsp ground ginger
115 g/4 oz caster sugar
85 g/3 oz margarine
4 tbsp golden syrup – measure with a warmed spoon
1 egg, beaten

Heat the oven to 180°C/350°F/gas 4. Grease four baking sheets.

Sift together the flour, baking powder, salt and ground ginger. Stir in the sugar. Melt the margarine and golden syrup together and add to the dry ingredients with the beaten egg. Mix together well.

Place small teaspoonfuls of the mixture in mounds on the baking sheets.

Bake in the centre of the oven for about 15 minutes. Leave to cool slightly, then transfer to a wire rack.

NUTTY SQUARES

Makes 24
Each square: 100 Cals/420 kJ, 1 g fibre

115 g/4 oz margarine
200 g/7 oz gluten-free rolled (porridge) oats
60 g/2 oz raisins or sultanas
60 g/2 oz demerara sugar
60 g/2 oz chopped peanuts (not salted)
1 egg, beaten

Heat the oven to 180°C/350°F/gas 4. Grease a 28 x 18-cm/11 x 7-in shallow tin and line with greased greaseproof paper. Melt the margarine. Mix all the dry ingredients in a large bowl, add the beaten egg and then the melted margarine. Mix well. Press firmly into the tin. Bake for 40-45 minutes or until well browned. Mark into squares while warm. Cool in the tin. Store in an airtight tin.

DATE AND NUT SQUARES

Makes 15
Each square: 140 Cals/590 kJ, 3 g fibre

85 g/3 oz hard margarine
115 g/4 oz stoned dates, chopped
60 g/2 oz soft brown sugar
30 g/1 oz walnuts, chopped
30 g/1 oz glacé cherries, chopped
60 g/2 oz Rice Krispies
30 g/1 oz soya bran
115 g/4 oz gluten-free plain chocolate

Grease an 18-cm/7-in square cake tin and line the bottom with greased greaseproof paper.

Place the margarine and the dates in a pan and heat slowly. Stir in the sugar and cook for a few minutes. Mix in the walnuts, cherries, Rice Krispies and bran. Press the mixture firmly into the prepared tin. Melt the chocolate in a basin over hot water, allow to cool slightly and spread over the biscuit mixture. Chill in the refrigerator until set. Cut into fingers.

PEANUT FINGERS

Makes 12
Each biscuit: 120 Cals/500 kJ, 2 g fibre

60 g/2 oz soft margarine
60 g/2 oz brown sugar
1 egg, beaten
½ tsp gluten-free baking powder
¼ tsp ground cinnamon
85 g/3 oz plain gluten-free flour
30 g/1 oz soya bran
60 g/2 oz gluten-free salted peanuts
milk to mix, as necessary

Heat the oven to 180°C/350°F/gas 4. Grease an 18-cm/7-in square tin.

Cream the margarine and sugar until light and fluffy. Beat the egg and blend into the creamed mixture. Sift the baking powder, cinnamon and flour together and fold into the mixture. Add the bran, the peanuts and a little milk if the mixture is too dry. Spread in the prepared tin and bake on the middle shelf until well browned, 20–30 minutes. Mark into fingers and leave to cool. Turn on to a wire rack while still warm. When cold store in an airtight tin; they will keep for about a week.

CHOCOLATE NUT FINGERS

Makes 24
Each finger: 130 Cals/550 kJ, 1 g fibre

170 g/6 oz plain gluten-free chocolate
115 g/4 oz walnuts, coarsely chopped
60 g/2 oz margarine
115 g/4 oz desiccated coconut
85 g/3 oz caster sugar
grated rind ½ orange
1 egg

Heat the oven to 180°C/350°F/gas 4. Grease a Swiss roll tin (28 x 18 cm/11 x 7 in and at least 2 cm/1 in deep) and line the base with a strip of greaseproof paper.

Break the chocolate into pieces and melt in a heatproof bowl over a pan of hot water. Stir in the chopped nuts. Spread the chocolate nut mixture evenly over the base of the tin. Leave to cool. Put the remaining ingredients into a bowl and beat until the mixture forms a smooth paste. Spread evenly over the chocolate. Bake for 25 minutes or until golden brown. Leave until cold and then cut into slim fingers.

FLORENTINES

Makes 24

Each biscuit: 80 Cals/340 kJ, 1 g fibre

60 g/2 oz butter
60 g/2 oz granulated sugar
2 tsp whipping cream
30 g/1 oz glacé cherries, chopped
30 g/1 oz chopped mixed peel
60 g/2 oz almonds, finely chopped
60 g/2 oz almonds, flaked
115 g/4 oz gluten-free plain chocolate

Heat the oven to 180°C/350°F/gas 4. Cover two large baking sheets with non-stick baking paper.

Melt the butter and sugar in a saucepan. Stir in the cream and remove from the heat. Blend in the rest of the ingredients except the chocolate. Place teaspoonfuls of the mixture well apart on the prepared baking sheets. Bake for 10–15 minutes or until golden brown. Melt the chocolate in a basin over hot water. When the biscuits are cold turn them over and spread the underside of each biscuit with a teaspoonful of chocolate. Leave to harden and store in an airtight tin.

BRANDY SNAPS

Makes 20

Each snap: 90 Cals/380 kJ, 0 g fibre

2 tbsp golden syrup – measure with a warmed spoon
60 g/2 oz hard margarine
60 g/2 oz granulated sugar
60 g/2 oz plain gluten-free flour
½ tsp ground ginger
1 tsp brandy or rum essence
225 ml/8 fl oz whipping cream, whipped until stiff

Heat the oven to 170°C/325°F/gas 3. Grease several baking sheets well. Put the golden syrup, margarine and sugar in a pan and heat gently. Stir until the sugar has dissolved and the margarine is melted – do not boil. Sift together the flour and ginger and beat into the syrup until smooth. Stir in the brandy or rum essence. Place 4–6 heaped teaspoonfuls, well spaced, on to each baking sheet. Bake one sheet at a time for 10 minutes each, turning the sheet round after 5 minutes to ensure even cooking. When the biscuits are golden brown, remove the tray and allow to cool for about 30 seconds. When the biscuits are just beginning to set, lift them with a palette knife and fold over the greased handle of a wooden spoon. Mould round the handle and rest on the baking sheet to cool. Slip the curled brandy snaps on to a cooling tray. If the biscuits set too quickly, return to the oven for a minute or two to soften and try again. After a little practice it is quite simple – using two wooden spoons makes it easier. Fill with whipped cream to serve but store unfilled in an airtight tin.

NB Brandy snaps are difficult to make but can be perfected with practice. This recipe makes excellent very thin, crisp snaps; here are some points to aid success.

- The baking sheets must be very well greased – use margarine or oil.
- Measure the ingredients very carefully, especially the syrup if you are making a smaller quantity.
- At first, bake just two snaps at a time for better, quicker removal from the baking sheet. As you become more skilled you can bake up to four at a time.

Melting moments

Makes 20
Each biscuit: 70 Cals/290 kJ, 0 g fibre

115 g/4 oz hard margarine
45 g/1½ oz icing sugar
60 g/2 oz self-raising gluten-free flour*
60 g/2 oz cornflour
3–4 drops vanilla essence

Heat the oven to 170°C/325°F/gas 3. Cover two baking sheets with greased greaseproof paper or non-stick baking paper.

Cream the margarine with the sugar until very light. Sift the flours together and work into the creamed mixture with the vanilla essence until very smooth. Pipe small biscuits on to the prepared sheets or, with gluten-free floured hands, form walnut-sized pieces into balls and flatten slightly with the back of a fork. Bake for about 20 minutes until pale gold. Allow to cool on a wire rack. Store in an airtight tin.

Alternatives
Sandwich together with a thick butter icing.

Add a few drops of very strong coffee to the mixture and sandwich with the coffee-flavoured cream icing.

For Viennese biscuits, pipe the mixture in swirls and decorate with a piece of glacé cherry.

* Tested with Juvela gluten-free mix

Coconut squares

Makes 9
Each square: 230 Cals/970 kJ, 2 g fibre

60 g/2 oz soft margarine
30 g/1 oz granulated sugar
1 egg
85 g/3 oz plain gluten-free flour
pinch salt
30 g/1 oz soya bran
2 tbsp raspberry jam
Topping:
85 g/3 oz desiccated coconut
85 g/3 oz granulated sugar
1 egg

Heat the oven to 180°C/350°F/gas 4. Grease an 18-cm/7-in square tin and line with greaseproof paper.

Cream the margarine and sugar until light and fluffy. Beat in the egg. Sift the flour and salt together and mix in. Stir in the bran. Spread this mixture over the base of the prepared tin. Warm the jam and spread on top. Mix the topping ingredients in a small bowl, spread on top of the jam, and mark the top lightly with a fork. Bake for 30–40 minutes or until lightly browned and firm. Leave to cool in the tin, then cut into squares. Store in a cool place.

Coconut and cherry chocolate slices

Makes 12
Each slice: 210 Cals/880 kJ, 2 g fibre

85 g/3 oz soft margarine
60 g/2 oz granulated sugar
1 egg
115 g/4 oz desiccated coconut
30 g/1 oz gluten-free flour
60 g/2 oz glacé cherries, chopped
115 g/4 oz gluten-free plain chocolate
15 g/½ oz margarine

Heat the oven to 180°C/350°F/gas 4. Grease an 18-cm/7-in square tin and line the bottom with greased greaseproof paper.

Cream the soft margarine and sugar until light. Beat in the egg. Mix the desiccated coconut with the flour and fold it in. Add the glacé cherries. Smooth into the prepared tin and bake for 20–30 minutes or until firm and brown. Leave in the tin to go cold. Melt the chocolate and 15 g/½ oz margarine in a small bowl placed over hot water, allow to cool and pour it over. As the chocolate sets mark with wavy lines with a fork and score into fingers. Store in a cool place.

Almond macaroons

Makes 15
Each macaroon: 50 Cals/210 kJ, 1 g fibre

1 egg white
70 g/2½ oz caster sugar
70 g/2½ oz ground almonds
2 drops almond essence

Heat the oven to 180°C/350°F/gas 4. Cover a baking sheet with non-stick baking paper.

Whisk the egg white until frothy but not too stiff. Fold in the sugar, ground almonds and essence. Take walnut-size pieces, roll quickly and lightly into balls (dip hands in cold water if the mixture becomes too sticky). Place on the baking sheet, leaving room for the macaroons to spread. Bake for 20–25 minutes or until pale golden. Allow to cool on the paper. Lift off when cold and store in an airtight container.

One tablespoonful of the ground almonds may be omitted and 1 tablespoonful ground rice used in its place.

SPICY DOUGHNUTS

Makes 9

Each doughnut: 350 Cals/1470 kJ, 0 g fibre

1 egg
115 g/4 oz granulated sugar
115 ml/4 fl oz milk
45 g/1½ oz margarine
340 g/12 oz plain gluten-free flour
2 tsp gluten-free baking powder
¼ tsp salt
¼ tsp ground cinnamon
¼ tsp ground nutmeg
olive oil for frying
For coating:
115 g/4 oz granulated sugar
1–2 tsp grated nutmeg

Put a sheet of absorbent paper on a baking sheet on which to drain the doughnuts. Mix 115 g/4 oz granulated sugar and 1–2 tsp grated nutmeg on a sheet of greaseproof paper. A fish slice and a carving fork are useful to slip the doughnuts into the oil and lift them out.

Beat the egg and whisk in the sugar and the milk. Melt the margarine and beat it in. Sift the dry ingredients together and fold into the egg and milk mixture. Mix to form a soft dough. Knead lightly to form a ball. Wrap in greaseproof paper and chill for 30 minutes until firm. Press the dough into a piece about 1 cm/½ in thick on a board dusted with gluten-free flour. Cut with a plain 5-cm/2-in cutter and use a 1-cm/½-in cutter to make a hole in the centre. Heat the oil in a deep-frying pan until hot. Test by dropping in a cube of gluten-free bread, which should brown in 30 seconds. Cook the doughnuts in the hot oil until light brown. Drain and turn in the sugar and nutmeg. Serve at once.

CHELSEA BUNS

Makes 8
Each bun: 230 Cals/950 kJ, 1 g fibre

250 g/9 oz Glutafin gluten-free white mix
5 g/½ sachet easy-blend dried yeast enclosed with mix
1 tsp gluten-free mixed spice
30 g/1 oz caster sugar
30 g/1 oz margarine
1 egg
60–75 ml/2–3 fl oz warm milk
30 g/1 oz butter or margarine
85 g/3 oz currants or raisins
30 g/1 oz soft brown sugar

Put the Glutafin mix, yeast, mixed spice and sugar in a bowl and mix together well. Rub in the margarine. Add the egg and enough of the warm milk to give a soft, but not sticky, dough. Turn on to a surface lightly dusted with Glutafin mix and knead until soft. Roll out to a 25 cm/10 in square. Melt the butter or margarine and brush over the dough. Sprinkle over the dried fruit and brown sugar and roll up firmly like a Swiss roll. Moisten the edge with water to seal. Cut into eight slices and place cut side down on a greased baking sheet. Cover with oiled polythene and leave to prove in a warm place for 20 minutes or until well risen. Heat the oven to 190°C/375°F/gas 5. Bake for 15–20 minutes until golden brown. Cool on a rack and then drizzle over glacé icing if desired.

Cakes

Cakes cooked with gluten-free flour turn out very well, but here are a few points to aid success. Check the cake 10 to 15 minutes before the final baking time: if it is browning too quickly, lower the temperature and/or cover it with greaseproof paper. To test if a fruit cake or teabread is cooked, push a skewer or knitting needle into the middle – when it is done the skewer will come out clean. To test a sponge cake, push the centre lightly with a finger and it should spring back. Leave all cakes in the tin for at least five minutes after cooking and then cool on a wire rack. If a cake cracks during baking it is usually because it is cooking too quickly.

Cakes are best frozen straight after baking and cooling. They can be decorated first (take care that the decorations are gluten-free) but keep longer if undecorated. Storage time for decorated cakes is four to six weeks, undecorated cakes about three months. Thaw cakes at room temperature. The thawing time depends on how thick the cake is – one hour for small cakes, two to three hours for larger cakes.

See also Baking and breadmaking, page 44, and Which flour to use?, page 52.

VICTORIA SANDWICH

Makes 10 slices
Each slice: 220 Cals/920 kJ, 0 g fibre

115 g/4 oz soft margarine
115 g/4 oz caster sugar
2 eggs
¼ tsp vanilla essence (optional)
115 g/4 oz plain gluten-free flour
pinch salt
½ tsp gluten-free baking powder
a little milk
jam
whipped cream

Heat the oven to 190°C/375°F/gas 5. Grease two 18-cm/7-in sandwich tins and line the bottoms with greased greaseproof paper.

Cream the margarine and sugar together, beat in the eggs one at a time and add the vanilla essence, if using. Sift the flour, salt and baking powder together into a bowl and fold into the creamed mixture, adding a little milk if necessary to make a soft-dropping consistency. Divide between the two tins and bake for about 20 minutes or until golden brown and firm. Cool on a wire rack. Sandwich together with jam and cream.

Alternatives
Use different flavourings, e.g. orange or lemon rind.

Add 60 g/2 oz mixed dried fruit and bake in prepared bun cases for 15–20 minutes. Makes about 12.

APPLE CAKE

Makes 8 slices
Each slice: 310 Cals/1300 kJ, 1 g fibre

140 g/5 oz soft margarine
85 g/3 oz granulated sugar
1 egg
200 g/7 oz plain gluten-free flour
½ tsp salt
½ tsp gluten-free baking powder
icing sugar, to decorate
Filling:
2 large cooking apples, peeled, cored and sliced
1 tsp ground cinnamon
85 g/3 oz granulated sugar

Heat the oven to 170°C/325°F/gas 3. Grease an 18-cm/7-in square tin or a 20-cm/8-in round tin and line with greaseproof paper.

Cream the margarine and sugar until light. Beat in the egg. Sift together the flour, salt and baking powder and fold into the mixture. Spread three-quarters on to the base of the prepared tin. Cover with the sliced apple and sprinkle with the cinnamon and sugar. Place teaspoonfuls of the remaining mixture on top. Bake in the centre of the oven until the cake is set and the apple is soft, about 1–1½ hours. Sprinkle with icing sugar and serve warm or cold as a dessert cake.

ALMOND CAKE

Makes 12 slices
Each slice: 220 Cals/920 kJ, 4 g fibre

115 g/4 oz blanched almonds
140 g/5 oz caster sugar
3 eggs
60 g/2 oz plain gluten-free flour
pinch salt
½ tsp gluten-free baking powder
45 g/1½ oz soya bran
85 g/3 oz margarine
1 tbsp kirsch or Amaretto liqueur

Heat the oven to 170°C/325°F/gas 3. Grease two 18–20-cm/7–8-in sandwich tins and line the bottoms with greased greaseproof paper.

Grind the almonds finely in a blender or food processor. Place the sugar and eggs in a large bowl and beat thoroughly until light and thick. Sift together the flour, salt and baking powder, add the bran and almonds and fold in lightly with a metal spoon. Melt the margarine. Fold the liqueur and margarine lightly into the batter. Pour into the two cake tins. Bake for 25–30 minutes or until the cake is firm. Cool for 5 minutes in the tin. Loosen the sides and turn gently on to a wire rack.

These cakes can be sandwiched together with apricot jam and dusted with icing sugar or served as a dessert with stewed apricots.

GOLDEN CAKE

Makes 10 slices
Each slice: 140 Cals/590 kJ, 1 g fibre

70 g/2½ oz gluten-free instant potato powder (not granules)
1 tsp gluten-free baking powder
85 g/3 oz margarine
4 tbsp golden syrup – measure with a warmed spoon
85 g/3 oz soft brown sugar
grated rind 1 orange
2 tbsp orange juice
2 eggs, separated
butter icing (optional)

Heat the oven to 180°C/350°F/gas 4. Grease a 16–18-cm/6–7-in sandwich tin and line it with greased greaseproof paper.

Place the instant potato and baking powder in a bowl and mix well. Heat the margarine, syrup, sugar, orange rind and juice in a pan, stirring to dissolve the sugar – do not boil. Pour the mixture on to the instant potato and beat well. Beat the egg yolks into the mixture. Whisk the egg whites until very stiff and lightly fold into the mixture. Pour into the tin and bake for 35–45 minutes. If browning too quickly, cover with a sheet of greaseproof paper after 30 minutes. Cool in the tin for 5 minutes then remove to a wire rack. When cold, store in an airtight tin in a cool place. Ice with butter icing if desired. Best eaten within two days.

MARMALADE CAKE

Makes 16 slices
Each slice: 160 Cals/670 kJ, 0 g fibre

115 g/4 oz soft margarine
115 g/4 oz soft brown sugar
2 eggs
225 g/8 oz plain gluten-free flour
4 tbsp coarse-cut marmalade
1 tsp gluten-free baking powder
pinch salt
¼ tsp gluten-free mixed spice
30 g/1 oz chopped mixed peel
2 tbsp milk to mix

Heat the oven to 170°C/325°F/gas 3. Grease a 450-g/1-lb loaf tin and line the bottom with greased greaseproof paper.

Cream the margarine and sugar very well, until light. Beat in the eggs one at a time with a teaspoonful of the flour. Add the marmalade and beat in. Sift the remaining flour, baking powder, salt and spice and fold in gradually. Mix in the peel and sufficient milk to form a fairly soft mixture. Spoon into the tin and bake in the middle of the oven for 1¼–1½ hours. If the cake browns too quickly, place a sheet of greaseproof paper over it. Leave to cool in the tin for 5 minutes. Lift out and cool on a wire rack. Keeps well stored in a cool place.

SEED CAKE

Makes 12 slices
Each slice: 90 Cals/380 kJ, 0 g fibre

85 g/3 oz soft margarine
85 g/3 oz granulated sugar plus extra for sprinkling
115 g/4 oz plain gluten-free flour
pinch salt
¼ tsp gluten-free baking powder
1 egg
30 g/1 oz chopped mixed peel
1½ tsp caraway seeds

Heat the oven to 180°C/350°F/gas 4. Grease an 18-cm/7-in sandwich tin and line the bottom with greased greaseproof paper.

Cream together the margarine and sugar. Sift together the flour, salt and baking powder. Beat the egg and add to the creamed mixture. Fold in the flour and add the peel and 1 teaspoonful caraway seeds. If the mixture is too stiff add a little cold milk, to form a soft dropping consistency. Spoon into the tin and level. Sprinkle extra sugar and seeds on top. Bake for 35–45 minutes or until firm and lightly browned.

SWISS ROLL

Makes 8 slices
Each slice: 110 Cals/460 kJ, 0 g fibre

3 eggs
85 g/3 oz caster sugar
85 g/3 oz Glutafin gluten-free white mix
warm jam
icing sugar

Heat the oven to 200°C/400°F/gas 6. Line a Swiss roll tin (18 x 28cm/ 7 x 11 in) with greased greaseproof paper.

Whisk together the eggs and sugar until thick, creamy and almost white in colour. The mixture should leave a trail when the whisk is removed. Lightly fold in the Glutafin mix. Pour the mixture into the prepared tin and bake for 10 minutes. It is a thin cake and bakes quickly. Do not overbake or the Swiss roll will crack. Have ready a sheet of greaseproof paper with sugar sprinkled on it. Turn the cake over quickly on to the paper. If the edges are crisp, trim them off. Spread with the warm jam. Roll up the cake, using the paper to help and keeping the roll as tight as possible. Leave to cool, resting on the seam. Dust with icing sugar.

Alternatives

For a chocolate Swiss roll, substitute 1 tablespoonful gluten-free cocoa for 1 tablespoonful of the gluten-free flour. Sift the remaining flour and cocoa together and proceed as before.

To fill with whipped cream or butter cream: roll the cake up while warm with a sheet of greaseproof paper inside. Cool. When cold unroll very gently and spread with the chosen filling. Re-roll, but not too tightly.

Cover with gluten-free chocolate butter cream to make a chocolate log for Christmas.

CHOCOLATE CAKE

Makes 12 slices
Each slice: 210 Cals/880 kJ, 0 g fibre

115 g/4 oz soft margarine
140 g/5 oz caster sugar
2 eggs
115 g/4 oz plain gluten-free flour
a few drops vanilla essence
pinch salt
1 tsp gluten-free baking powder
30 g/1 oz gluten-free cocoa

Heat the oven to 180°C/350°F/gas 4. Grease two 18-cm/7-in sandwich tins and line the bottoms with greased greaseproof paper.

Cream the margarine and sugar together until light. Beat in the eggs one at a time, adding a little flour if necessary to prevent curdling. Add the vanilla essence and fold in the rest of the flour sifted together with the salt, baking powder and cocoa. Divide the mixture between the two tins and bake for 25–35 minutes or until firm. Remove the cakes from the tins and cool on wire racks.

These cakes can be served separately or sandwiched together with whipped cream, butter cream or jam. They can be iced with chocolate or coffee icing.

CHOCOLATE PARCEL CAKE

Serves 8–10

Each slice: 400 Cals/1660 kJ, 1 g fibre

225 g/8 oz Glutafin mix
2 level tsp bicarbonate of soda
60 g/2 oz caster sugar
115 g/4 oz soft margarine
2 eggs
1 tbsp lemon juice
225 ml/8 fl oz milk
Fudge icing:
30 g/1 oz margarine or butter
30 g/1 oz gluten-free cocoa*
170 g/6 oz icing sugar
about 1½ tbsp milk
Decoration:
2 m/2 yd ribbon
chocolate leaves or shapes* (optional)

Heat the oven to 180°C/350°F/gas 4. Line an 18-cm/7-in square cake tin with non-stick baking paper.

Put all the ingredients for the cake into a large bowl and mix well. Pour into the tin and bake for 40–50 minutes, until the cake springs back when touched. Leave to cool.

Make the icing by melting the margarine or butter. Add the cocoa, stir well and then stir in the icing sugar and milk.

When the cake is cool, pour the icing over the top of the cake and spread out evenly. Leave to set. Tie a ribbon over the cake to make it look like a parcel. Decorate with chocolate leaves or shapes if desired.

* Check in your Coeliac UK *Directory*, under *Drinks* and *Ingredients: cake decorations*, for allowable makes.

CHOCOLATE MUNCHY CAKE

Makes 12 slices
Each slice: 190 Cals/800 kJ, 2 g fibre

115 g/4 oz plain gluten-free chocolate
85 g/3 oz margarine
1 egg yolk, beaten
115 g/4 oz gluten-free digestive biscuits, crushed
60 g/2 oz raisins or sultanas
30 g/1 oz glacé cherries, chopped (optional)
60 g/2 oz flaked almonds, toasted

Grease a loose-bottomed flan or sandwich tin and line the bottom with greased greaseproof paper. Break the chocolate into pieces and place, with the margarine, in a basin over hot water to soften. Cool slightly. Add the egg to the chocolate mixture. Stir in the biscuit crumbs, fruit and nuts. Turn the mixture into the prepared tin and smooth the top. Mark top into slices when nearly set. Chill for at least 1 hour before serving.

CARROT CAKE

Makes 12 slices
Each slice: 230 Cals/970 kJ, 3 g fibre

6 eggs, separated
225 g/8 oz granulated sugar
225 g/8 oz ground almonds
¼ tsp ground cinnamon
30 g/1 oz ground rice
225 g/8 oz carrots, finely grated
grated rind 1 lemon
1–2 tbsp lemon juice

Heat the oven to 190°C/375°F/gas 5. Grease two 18-cm/7-in tins and line the bottoms with greased greaseproof paper.

Put the egg yolks in a bowl with the sugar and beat until light and creamy. Mix the ground almonds, cinnamon and ground rice together and blend well. Fold the almond mixture and carrots into the creamed mixture with the lemon rind and juice. Finally, beat the egg whites until stiff and fold them in very lightly to form a soft dropping consistency. Pour the batter into the two tins and bake for 20 minutes. Reduce the oven temperature to 180°C/350°F/gas 4 if the cakes are browning too quickly, and bake for a further 20–25 minutes. Remove from the tins and cool on a wire tray. Keep in a refrigerator.

A dessert cake. Can be sandwiched together with apricot jam and served with tinned or stewed apricots or peaches.

GINGER CAKE

Makes 16 slices
Each slice: 180 Cals/760 kJ, 1 g fibre

340 g/12 oz plain gluten-free flour
½ tsp gluten-free baking powder
pinch salt
½ tsp ground ginger
30 g/1 oz soya bran
115 g/4 oz butter or margarine
115 g/4 oz granulated sugar plus a little for sprinkling
2 eggs
115 g/4 oz preserved ginger, drained and chopped
milk to mix, as necessary

Heat the oven to 180°C/350°F/gas 4. Grease an 18-cm/7-in round tin or a large 1-kg/2-lb loaf tin and line the bottom with greased greaseproof paper.

Sift together the flour, baking powder, salt and ginger and mix in the bran. Cream together the butter or margarine and sugar and beat in the eggs, one at a time. Fold in the dry ingredients together with the chopped ginger. Add about 5 tablespoonfuls milk. The mixture should drop off the spoon when shaken gently. Pour into the prepared tin. Sprinkle sugar over the top. Bake for 1¼–1½ hours or until well risen, brown and firm. Cool on a wire rack. Wrap in foil and store in an airtight tin. This cake keeps for a week or two.

STICKY GINGERBREAD

Makes 12 squares
Each square: 240 Cals/1010 kJ, 0 g fibre

225 g/8 oz Glutafin gluten-free white mix
pinch salt
2 tsp ground ginger
1 tsp gluten-free mixed spice
1 tsp bicarbonate of soda
60 g/2 oz soft brown sugar
115 g/4 oz margarine
6 tbsp black treacle – measure with a warmed spoon
2 tbsp golden syrup – measure with a warmed spoon
140 ml/5 fl oz milk
2 eggs, beaten

Heat the oven to 150°C/300°F/gas 2. Grease a 15 x 23-cm/6 x 9-in cake tin and line the bottom with greased greaseproof paper.

Sift together the flour, salt, ginger, mixed spice and bicarbonate of soda. Stir in the sugar. Melt the margarine, treacle and syrup gently together. Gradually beat in the milk. Allow to cool and add the eggs. Stir the treacle mixture into the dry ingredients. Pour into the cake tin and bake for about 45–50 minutes.

PARKIN

Makes 12 pieces
Each piece: 140 Cals/590 kJ, 7 g fibre

115 g/4 oz soya bran
60 g/2 oz plain gluten-free flour
1 tsp gluten-free baking powder
1 tsp ground ginger
60 g/2 oz hard margarine
60 g/2 oz brown sugar
2 tbsp black treacle – measure with a warmed spoon
5 tbsp golden syrup – measure with a warmed spoon
1 egg, beaten

Heat the oven to 170°C/325°F/gas 3. Grease an 18-cm/7-in square shallow tin and line with greaseproof paper.

Mix together the soya bran, flour, baking powder and ginger. Melt the margarine over a low heat and add the sugar, treacle and syrup, stirring until the sugar is dissolved. Add to the dry ingredients with the egg. Mix to a batter that drops easily from the spoon. Pour into the prepared tin and bake for about 45 minutes or until firm. When cool wrap in foil and, ideally, keep for a few days before eating. Keeps well stored in a cool place.

BOILED FRUIT CAKE

Makes 16 slices
Each slice: 150 Cals/630 kJ, 1 g fibre

140 g/5 oz dark brown sugar or molasses sugar
140 ml/5 fl oz milk
60 g/2 oz margarine
85 g/3 oz dried mixed fruit
115 g/4 oz ground rice
85 g/3 oz cornmeal
85 g/3 oz soya flour
1 tsp gluten-free mixed spice
1 tsp gluten-free baking powder
1 egg, beaten

Heat the oven to 180°C/350°F/gas 4. Grease a 1-kg/2-lb loaf tin.

Heat the sugar, milk, margarine and dried fruit together in a pan but do not boil. Stir until the sugar is dissolved, then leave to cool slightly. Sift all the dry ingredients together into a bowl. Add the fruit mixture and the egg. Mix well. Spoon into the greased loaf tin and level the mixture. Bake on the middle shelf for about 40 minutes. If it is browning too quickly, lower the heat to 170°C/325°F/gas 3. Cool in the tin. This cake keeps well, stored in an airtight tin.

Rich fruit cake

Makes 16 slices
Each slice: 250 Cals/1050 kJ, 2 g fibre

140 g/5 oz hard margarine
140 g/5 oz soft brown sugar
2 tsp black treacle – measure with a warmed spoon
225 g/8 oz plain gluten-free flour
½ tsp gluten-free baking powder
1 tsp gluten-free mixed spice
3 eggs
340 g/12 oz mixed dried fruit
85 g/3 oz glacé cherries, chopped
60 g/2 oz ground almonds
2–4 tbsp milk

Heat the oven to 170°C/325°F/gas 3. Grease and line with two layers of greaseproof paper an 18-cm/7-in square cake tin or 20-cm/8-in round cake tin.

Cream the margarine, sugar and treacle until soft. Sift together the flour, baking powder and mixed spice. Beat in the eggs one at a time with a teaspoonful of flour, beating well each time. Fold in half the sifted flour. Then fold in the dried fruit and chopped cherries mixed with the rest of the flour and the ground almonds. The mixture should be of a heavy dropping consistency – if it is too stiff add 2–4 tablespoonfuls milk. Spoon into the prepared tin and bake for 1½ hours in the middle of the oven. Then lower the oven temperature to 150°C/300°F/gas 2, cover the top with two sheets of greaseproof paper and cook for a further 1–1½ hours, until a skewer comes out clean. Cool on a wire rack and when cold wrap, with its greaseproof paper, in foil. Store in a cool place. Allow several days at least to mature.

If this cake is to be used as a Christmas cake, bake with butter and keep for one month well wrapped and stored in a cool place. One week before the cake is required, unwrap and turn it upside down. Prick the bottom and dribble brandy into it. Cover with gluten-free marzipan and ice.

Sauces

Tinned, packet or bottled sauces, gravy mixes and brownings may contain gluten. Use cornflour to thicken. Many recipes use cornflour anyway; but if you are substituting it for ordinary flour you will need about two-thirds as much.

WHITE SAUCE

Total: 350 Cals/1470 kJ, 0 g fibre

4 tsp cornflour
285 ml/½ pt milk
knob of margarine
salt and freshly ground black pepper

In a basin, blend the cornflour to a smooth cream with a little milk. Heat the remaining milk with the margarine until boiling and pour on to the cornflour, stirring well. Return the mixture to the pan and bring to the boil, stirring continuously with a wooden spoon. Simmer for 1–2 minutes. Season to taste. If making one of the variations below, stir in the extra ingredients and heat through.

Cheese sauce

Total: 590 Cals/2480 kJ, 0 g fibre

60 g/2 oz grated cheese
¼ tsp gluten-free prepared mustard

Mushroom sauce

Total: 480 Cals/2020 kJ, 0 g fibre

60 g/2 oz mushrooms, finely sliced and fried

Parsley sauce

Total: 350 Cals/1470 kJ, 0 g fibre

½ tbsp finely chopped fresh parsley

FRESH TOMATO SAUCE

Total: 1150 Cals/4830 kJ, 9 g fibre

4 tbsp olive oil
1 medium onion, very finely chopped
60 g/2 oz bacon, diced
1 clove garlic, crushed (optional)
1 small carrot, chopped
340 g/12 oz tomatoes, skinned and chopped
4 tbsp gluten-free tomato purée
170 ml/6 fl oz gluten-free stock or water
2 tbsp cornflour
1 bay leaf
2 cloves
4 black peppercorns
pinch dried basil
1 tbsp brown sugar
½ tsp salt
3 tsp lemon juice

Heat the oil in a large heavy saucepan. Add the onion, bacon, garlic (if using) and carrot. Cover the pan and fry gently for about 6 minutes. Shake the pan frequently to prevent sticking. Stir in the tomatoes and the tomato purée. Add the stock or water. Blend the cornflour with a little cold water and add to the mixture. Cook, stirring continuously, until the sauce boils and thickens. Add the rest of the ingredients. Cover and simmer for about 40 minutes, stirring frequently. Sieve the sauce, taste and adjust the seasoning.

Serve hot or cold. Store in a screw-top jar in the refrigerator.

SPANISH SAUCE

Each 15 ml tablespoon: 120 Cals/460 kJ, 0 g fibre

1 quantity gluten-free Mayonnaise (page 63)
4 tbsp gluten-free tomato purée
4 tbsp finely chopped pimento
salt and freshly ground black pepper

Combine all the ingredients. Store in the refrigerator.

Quick tomato sauce

Total: 420 Cals/1760 kJ, 3 g fibre

30 g/1 oz margarine
1 small onion, grated
1 small apple, peeled and grated
6 tbsp gluten-free tomato purée
salt and freshly ground black pepper
¼ tsp sugar
2 tsp cornflour
285 ml/½ pt water

Melt the margarine in a pan and fry the onion and apple for a few minutes until soft. Add the tomato purée, seasoning and sugar. Blend the cornflour with a little water to make a smooth cream and stir into the mixture in the pan. Finally, add the remaining water and bring to the boil, stirring continuously until smooth and thick. Simmer gently for about 10 minutes. Adjust the seasoning. Serve warm.

Barbecue sauce

Total: 730 Cals/3070 kJ, 1 g fibre

60 g/2 oz margarine
1 medium onion, finely chopped
1 clove garlic, crushed
1 tbsp prepared gluten-free English mustard
2 tbsp vinegar
large pinch gluten-free cayenne pepper
2 tbsp brown sugar
1 thick slice lemon
4 tbsp gluten-free tomato purée
2 tbsp Worcestershire sauce

Melt the margarine in a small saucepan and fry the onion and garlic for a few minutes, until soft but not brown. Stir in the mustard, vinegar, cayenne pepper, sugar, lemon and 140 ml/5 fl oz water. Bring to the boil and simmer for 15 minutes, stirring occasionally. Add the tomato purée and Worcestershire sauce, stir and simmer for another 5 minutes. Remove the lemon and serve.

TARTARE SAUCE

Each 15 ml tablespoon: 100 Cals/420 kJ, 0 g fibre

1 quantity gluten-free Mayonnaise (page 63)
1 tbsp chopped fresh parsley
4 tbsp capers, finely chopped
4 tbsp gherkins, finely chopped

Mix all the ingredients together. Store in the refrigerator.

CURRY SAUCE

Total: 830 Cals/3490 kJ, 20 g fibre

1 tbsp olive oil
1 onion, finely chopped
1 clove garlic, crushed
1½ tsp cornflour
4–6 tbsp gluten-free curry powder
285 ml/½ pt gluten-free stock or water
1 small apple, coarsely grated
30–60 g/1–2 oz desiccated coconut (optional)
1 tbsp currants (optional)
1 tbsp lemon juice
salt and freshly ground black pepper
60 ml/2 fl oz top of the milk

Heat the oil in a saucepan and fry the onion and garlic for a few
minutes, until soft but not brown. Sprinkle in the cornflour and curry
powder, stir, and cook for a little longer. Gradually blend in the stock
or water, and, stirring continuously, bring to the boil. Cover and
simmer for about 20 minutes, stirring occasionally. Add the apple,
coconut and currants, if using, lemon juice and seasoning, stir in the
top of the milk and heat through.

Useful Addresses

Coeliac UK
P.O. Box No 220
High Wycombe
Bucks
HP11 2HY
Helpline: 0870 4448804
Website: www.coeliac.co.uk
Email: admin@coeliac.co.uk
Coeliac UK is an excellent source for further information – they have a good section of frequently asked questions ranging from the gum on postage stamps to buckwheat.

Food Standards Agency
Aviation House
125 Kingsway
London
WC2B 6NH
Tel: 020 7276 8000
Website: www.foodstandards.gov.uk

General Dietary Ltd
P.O. Box 38
Kingston-upon-Thames
Surrey
KT2 7YP
Tel: 020 8336 2323

Gluten-Free Foods Ltd
Tel: 0208 953 4444
Website: www.glutenfree-foods.co.uk

Juvela
The Juvela Nutrition Centre
100 Wavertree Boulevard
Liverpool
L7 9PT
Tel/Advice Line: 0151 228 1992
Website: www.juvela.co.uk
Email: juvela@shsint.co.uk

Larkhall Green Farm
225 Putney Bridge Road
London
SW15 2PY
Tel: 0181 874 1130
Fax: 0181 871 0066

National Osteoporosis Society
Camerton
Bath
BA2 0PJ
Tel: 01761 471771 (for general enquiries)
Helpline: 0845 4500230 (for medical queries)
Fax: 01761 471104
E-mail: info@nos.org.uk
Website: www.nos.org.uk

Nutricia Dietary Care
Newmarket Avenue
White Horse Business Park
Trowbridge
Wiltshire
BA14 0XQ
Tel/Advice Line: 01225 711801
Fax: 01225 711567
Websites: www.glutafin.co.uk *and* www.trufree.co.uk
E-mail: glutenfree@nutricia.co.uk

Nutrition Point Ltd
13 Taurus Park
Westbrook
Warrington
WA5 7ZT
Tel: 0704 154 4044
Website: www.nutritionpoint.co.uk
E-mail: info@nutritionpoint.co.uk

Scientific Hospital Supplies Ltd
100 Wavertree Road Boulevard
Wavertree Technology Park
Liverpool
L7 9PT
Tel: 0151 228 1992

Ultrapharm Ltd
P.O. Box 18
Henley on Thames
RG9 2AW
Tel: 01491 578016
Website: www.gfdiet.com

The Vegetarian Society
Parkdale
Dunham Road
Altrincham
Cheshire
WA14 4QG
Tel: 0161 925 2000
Website: www.vegsoc.org

INTERNATIONAL COELIAC GROUPS
exist in many countries and can
easily be found via listings on the
internet – for example at:

http://www.coeliac.co.uk/links/
international.htm

http://www.enabling.org/ia/celiac/
groups/groupsin.html#index

http://celiac.spb.ru/www.htm

Coeliac UK will also supply contact
details for other groups by telephone,
or by post if you send a stamped
addressed envelope.

Index